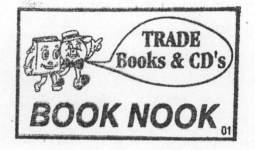

T'ai Chi Ch'uan
for Health and Self-Defense

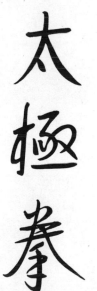

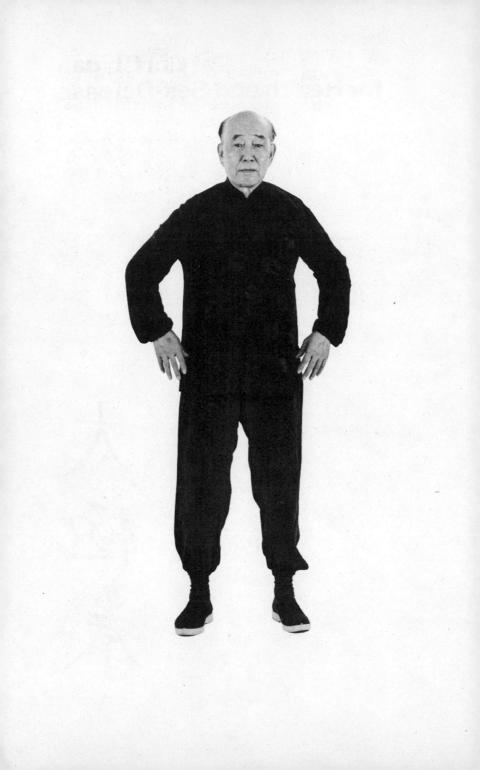

T'ai Chi Ch'uan

For Health and Self-Defense

Philosophy and Practice

Master T.T. Liang

Edited and with a Foreword by Paul B. Gallagher

Revised, expanded edition

Vintage Books
A Division of Random House
New York

Library of Congress Cataloging in Publication Data

Liang, T. T.
T'ai chi ch'uan for health and self-defense.

1. T'ai chi ch'uan.   I.   Title.
GV505.L5 1977   796.8'159   77–76553
ISBN 0–394–72461–5

Cover photo: James R. Smith

Manufactured in the United States of America

B9

Foreword

T'ai Chi Ch'uan or "Supreme Ultimate Boxing" is one of the finest products of Chinese philosophy and culture. Based upon the principles of the *I Ching* and the philosophy of Lao Tze, T'ai Chi Ch'uan is a system of rounded, fluid, balanced movements to be practiced daily for health and peace of mind. When the movements have been mastered, one's intrinsic energy developed, and one's equilibrium stable, the movements and postures of T'ai Chi can be employed to neutralize aggressive actions directed at the self and to counterattack.

Clearly, this book is not intended as a "teach yourself" manual of T'ai Chi for the rank beginner, even though beginners can profit from studying many of the treatises in this book, particularly the translations of the T'ai Chi Ch'uan Classics and the "Ten Guiding Points." It is presumed that the reader will be acquainted with the rudimentary facts about T'ai Chi —that the complete "long style" sequence of movements consists of 81, 108, 128, or 150 forms, depending upon the method used to count them; that all movements are relaxed and circular, directed by a calm yet concentrated mind; and that "oral guidance by a competent teacher" is required for anyone seriously interested in pursuing the study of this art.

Master T. T. Liang based his study and teaching of Yang Style T'ai Chi squarely upon the T'ai Chi Classics, a group of writings containing the fundamental principles of the art. The three major texts known collectively as Classics are the "T'ai Chi Ch'uan Classic," attributed to founder Chang San Feng of the late Sung Dynasty; the "Treatise on T'ai Chi Ch'uan," attributed to Wang Chung Yueh of the Ming Dynasty; and the "Mental Elucidation of the Thirteen Postures," also attributed to Wang Chung Yueh. These Classics appear in this book, translated in their entirety with a detailed original commentary by Master Liang. In this age of rapidly proliferating books on T'ai Chi, many of which contain not even a reference to the Classics, the translations here will provide a basis for correct study. The commentaries are especially valuable, and to my knowledge this is the first time that such detailed commentaries on the Classics have appeared in English. Because of the increasing popularity of T'ai Chi, Master Liang is especially anxious that students should base their study and practice upon the principles in the Classics, for the Classics are the indispensible foundation of the art. In proportion as one's practice deviates from the principles in the Classics, one will fall short of attaining the true meaning and function of T'ai Chi.

In addition to the three major Classics there is an extensive literature on T'ai Chi available to readers of Chinese. There are numerous essays, "songs," poems, and aphorisms expressing principles of T'ai Chi practice, either for health or self-defense. In Chinese books on T'ai Chi one can also find a variety of stories dealing with the exploits of famous masters. Several such tales are included in this volume to give students the flavor of this area of T'ai Chi literature. Though some of the stories, such as the story of the swallow landing on the master's hand, are well known and quite possibly grounded in fact, others tend toward what the Chinese call "wild history." May the reader enjoy them, but not expect perfect factual accuracy.

Since few of the above-mentioned essays and songs have yet

appeared in English, Master Liang hopes that this book will be a first step toward making some of this literature available to English-speaking people. However, many of the essays are terse and quite abstruse, so that even in Chinese books the original text is frequently elucidated in a commentary written by an experienced master. As Master Liang frequently said, unless one had acquired comprehension of the principles by practicing the art over a long period of time, he could not hope to understand the deepest meaning of the essays and Classics, many of which were written by former masters as an expression of their own profound comprehension of the principles of T'ai Chi. Thus a mere translation does not suffice; the translator himself must have sufficiently ripened in T'ai Chi practice to discern the true meaning of the texts. Master Liang's experience speaks for itself and his fine command of English makes these translations possible.

To date, few T'ai Chi books in English have gone beyond the requirements of the beginner in learning the movements of the solo form sequence. Master Liang intended that this small book would be suitable for students who had learned the entire sequence of movements and wished to further their knowledge by beginning the study of the Pushing Hands exercises. Many of the texts, therefore, apply specifically to techniques and principles studied in Pushing Hands practice.

The Pushing Hands exercise consists of two partners executing the movements of Ward Off, Roll Back, Press, and Push (the first four of the eight Postures) in circular alternations. The remaining four movements, Pull, Split, Elbow-Stroke, and Shoulder-Stroke, are practiced in a more advanced form of two-man exercise called Ta Lü. Both of these exercises, as the texts indicate, are intended to develop sensitivity to the movements and intentions of another and an intimate awareness of one's own state of balance at every moment. The partners gradually learn how to neutralize attacks and to discover each other's weak points for counterattacking. Pushing Hands and Ta Lü also teach the specific application and function of the eight basic movements.

The original texts were translated directly as they have come down to us. The commentaries on the Classics are Master Liang's own. The commentary on the "Song of Pushing Hands" is a translated commentary, modified frequently by Master Liang's own comments or observations. In a few places the interpretations given in this commentary differ from Master Liang's own way of teaching. Thus, there is a statement that one can at times entice an opponent to attack by using feints. This is in direct contrast to Master Liang's teaching in which he always emphasized that one should never take the initiative (i.e., make the first aggressive move). If the reader should discover any apparent inconsistencies in the texts, they may be taken as an indication of how different masters, at widely varying times and places, view the art in different ways, while not deviating from the central perspective provided by the Classics.

A few notes on matters covered in the translations may be in order for those readers not fully acquainted with the terminology in the texts. Tan t'ien is a Taoist term referring to a center of energy located approximately two inches below the navel. As one practices the movements, relaxing completely and breathing correctly without strain or roughness, energy gradually develops (i.e., "Ch'i sinks") in the tan t'ien and in time will circulate throughout the entire body. Literally tan t'ien means "Field of Cinnabar," another Taoist term referring to energies latent in man. The Field of Cinnabar is the place in which one can begin to produce the elixir of immortality.

The Five Elements or Agents of Chinese philosophy (Wood, Fire, Earth, Metal, Water) may be described as five stages of change or transformation in the continuing cosmic cycle; they may also be regarded as physical or metaphysical powers. Wood creates Fire, which creates Earth, which creates Metal, which creates Water, which creates Wood. The Elements can also subdue or conquer each other: Wood destroys Earth; Fire destroys Metal; Earth destroys Water; Metal destroys Wood; Water destroys Fire. In the context of T'ai Chi Ch'uan, "destroy" can mean neutralize. Thus, the different steps can be used to neutralize each other. However, in every movement, indeed at every moment in practice, one must maintain the condition of Central Equilibrium, symbolized in the diagram by the Element Earth. In this sense, for purposes of T'ai Chi practice, one can regard Earth as the fundamental Element.

In conclusion I would like to convey to the reader one of Master Liang's oft-repeated adages: "You should learn from many teachers, read many books. But only by serious practice can you discover the truth for yourself."

—Paul B. Gallagher
Wu Ming valley house
Season of Melting Snows
1977

The Five Elements

advance

gaze to left · central look to right
equilibrium

retreat

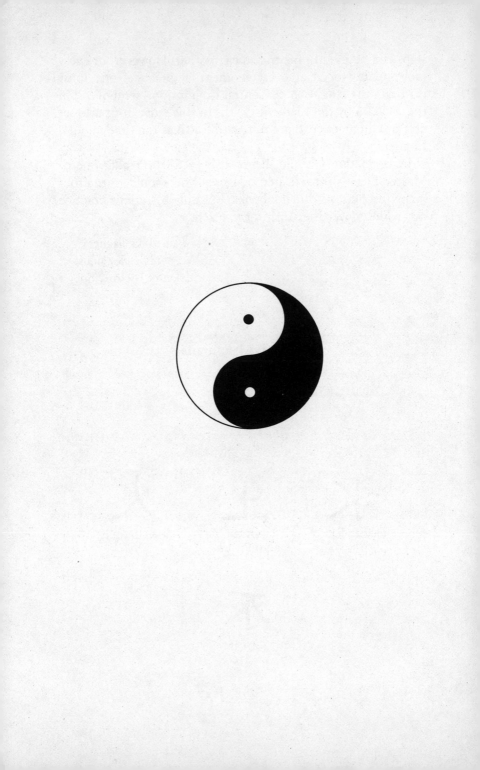

Acknowledgments

First, I would like to express the gratitude of all of Master Liang's students for the generosity of his teaching. This book commemorates his twelve years of teaching in this country; let us use it well.

Thanks are due to Dorothy Koval for her work with Master Liang's autobiographical sketch, his statement of general principles, and the several other texts in which she skillfully smoothed out the rough places.

Barbara Root is to be thanked for appearing in the photographs with Master Liang. The photos were taken by Benjamin Mendlowitz.

And thanks to all other friends who helped in ways large and small.

—P.B.G.

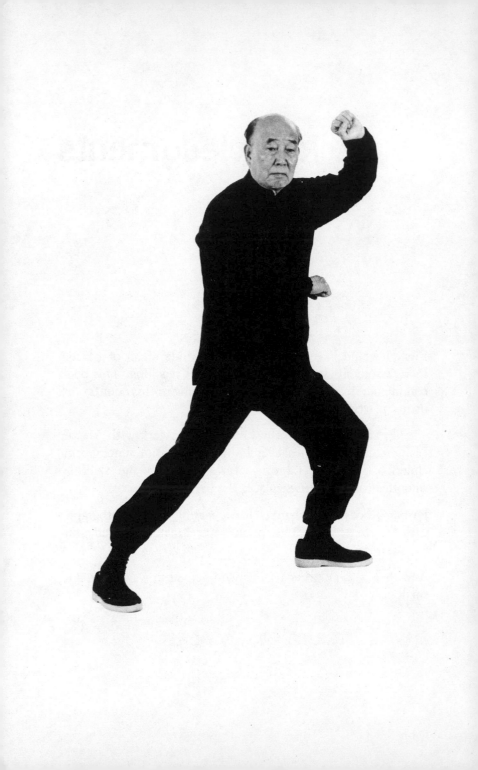

Contents

Foreword   v

Preface   xv

1 T'ai Chi Ch'uan and the Fundamental Principles   3

2 My Experience   7

3 My Personal View   11

4 The Complete Set of T'ai Chi Exercises   15

5 The T'ai Chi Classics
   T'ai Chi Ch'uan Classic   17
   The Mental Elucidation of the Thirteen Postures   22
   T'ai Chi Ch'uan Treatise   33
   Song of the Substance and Function of the Thirteen Postures   46

6 The Essentials of T'ai Chi Ch'uan   53

7 The Ten Guiding Points of T'ai Chi Ch'uan   61

8 Discussion of the Mind-Intent and the Ch'i   69

9 Slowness and Non-exertion of Muscular Force   73

10 Secrets (the Secret Technique) of the Eight Postures   77

11 Detailed Explanation of the Essential Meaning of the Five Elements   85

12 (T'ai Chi Ch'uan) Song of Pushing Hands,
   with Explanatory Comments   89
13 Other Short Texts   101
14 Stories of the Masters
   *The deflection of a thousand pound momentum by a
   trigger force of merely four ounces and an old man's
   defeating great numbers of young ones*   115
   A short biography of the Yang Family   118
   The secret bitterness of Yang Family T'ai Chi   124
15 Similar Philosophical Points: Lao Tze and
   T'ai Chi Ch'uan   131

Preface

At first I take up T'ai Chi as a hobby,
Gradually I become addicted to it,
Finally I can no longer get rid of it.
I must keep on practicing for my whole life—
    it is the only way to preserve health.
The more I practice, the more I want to learn
    from teachers and books.
The more I learn, the less I feel I know.
The theory and philosophy of T'ai Chi is so
    profound and abstruse!
I must continue studying forever and ever . . .
It is the only way to improve and better myself.

                             —T. T. Liang

T'ai Chi Ch'uan
for Health and Self-Defense

太
極
拳

1
T'ai Chi Ch'uan and the Fundamental Principles

T'ai Chi Ch'uan (commonly called T'ai Chi) is an ancient Chinese form of classical dance for health and self-defense created by a Taoist named Chang San-feng of the Sung Dynasty. There were originally 13 postures: Ward Off, Roll Back, Press, Push, Pull, Split, Elbow-Stroke, Shoulder-Stroke, Advance, Retreat, Gaze to Left, Look to Right, and Central Equilibrium.

The fundamental principles, which I quote from the T'ai Chi Classics, are: "To concentrate the ch'i"—an inherent oxygen in the body which gives stamina and vitality and ultimately brings one to the pliability of an infant—for health. It is said in the Classics that "When the lowest vertebrae are plumb erect, the spirit of vitality reaches the top of the head; when the top of the head feels as if suspended from above, the whole body will feel light and nimble." This is the way to strengthen the spine. By strengthening the spine, not only are the internal vital organs made strong, the brain is strengthened as well.

The Classics also say: "The ch'i sinks to the tan t'ien." When your ch'i sinks to the tan t'ien, your whole body will become relaxed and the blood will circulate freely through it unhindered.

The Classics say: "The ch'i should be stimulated." This stimulation of the ch'i can be compared to the small waves which form on a lake when the wind blows them to and fro in a system of troughs and crests. When the ch'i is stimulated in this way, it produces heat. Gradually this heat increases and penetrates the bones and becomes marrow. For example, although we do not see power in a glass of water, once it is turned into steam, it will drive the pistons of very powerful engines. Something has happened to it which makes it active and effective—its latent power has been released. After you have practiced in this way for a certain period, your health will be perfect —this is the way toward immortality.

When you have attained perfect health, we can proceed to discuss the second fundamental principle, namely, the practical use of T'ai Chi Ch'uan for self-defense. The proper application and functioning of T'ai Chi depends entirely on the player's consciousness: "the capacity to take advantage of your opponent's defects and to use your superior position." "To deflect the momentum of a thousand pounds with a trigger force of four ounces." "It is only from the greatest pliability and from yielding completely that you can attain power and ascendency." These sayings from the Classics emphasize mental activity rather than the use of external muscular force. You must pass through three processes before you can put the postures to practical use.

1. After practicing the 150 postures for a certain period of time, you will attain central equilibrium (a firm rooting of the feet); without this, your waist will not obey your orders and wishes.

2. You will learn how to yield (to neutralize the opponent's attacking force) without using resistance (force against force), through practicing the "Pushing Hands" exercise with a partner. Thus one must learn to lose, not gain—"small loss, small

gain: great loss, great gain." From Pushing Hands, you will learn the techniques of adhere, attach, connect, and follow, without letting go and with no resistance.

3. After you have learned how to yield completely, you will begin to learn how to counterattack. You will have to learn withdraw-and-attack techniques, folding techniques, how to find your opponent's defects and your own superior position, how to locate your opponent's center of gravity, how to concentrate on one point, how to avoid double-weighting, how to find the opponent's straight line, how to develop intrinsic energy (the energy which comes from the sinews and tendons) while avoiding the use of external muscular force (a force from the bones). By constant vigorous practice done correctly in this manner, plus study and remembering, one can reach the stage of total reliance on the mind. Go gradually, following the right method; above all, learn these techniques correctly. When you have all these techniques indelibly in your mind, counterattack is absolutely certain to be effective. If it is otherwise and these techniques are not in your mind, it will be a mere blind attack.

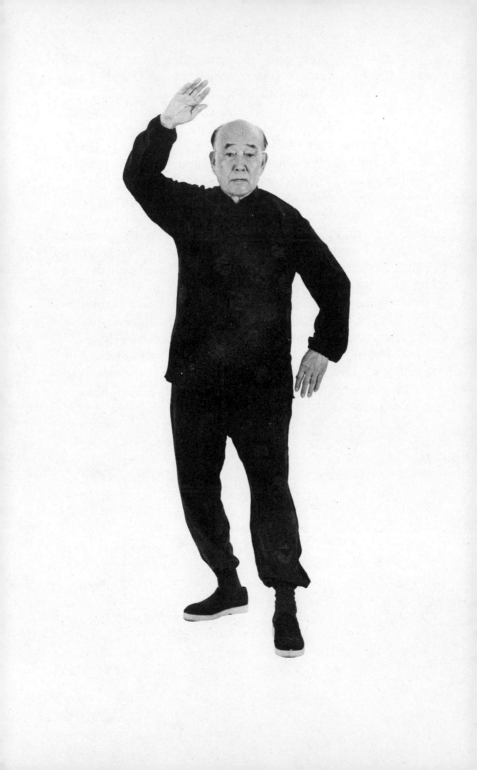

2
My Experience

I am nearing eighty years old and have been practicing T'ai Chi for more than thirty years. I, personally, have had fifteen teachers.

In the beginning I took up T'ai Chi in order to save my life after a very grave illness. At first I became involved because I was afraid that I might become ill again. As I got better and had further experience with T'ai Chi, I gradually became more and more interested in trying to make the art both more scientific and more esthetic. I introduced rhythm so that the postures can be practiced to music, slowly, effortlessly, and continuously. After sufficient practice, you will master the 150 postures so thoroughly that you will forget the rhythm, the movement, even yourself—although you are proceeding as usual. At this stage, you are in a trance; your five attributes (form, perception, consciousness, action, and knowledge) are all empty—this is meditation in action and action in meditation. When you finish and come to the end of the postures, suddenly you are back. Where have I been? What have I been doing? I don't know and I don't remember. This is complete

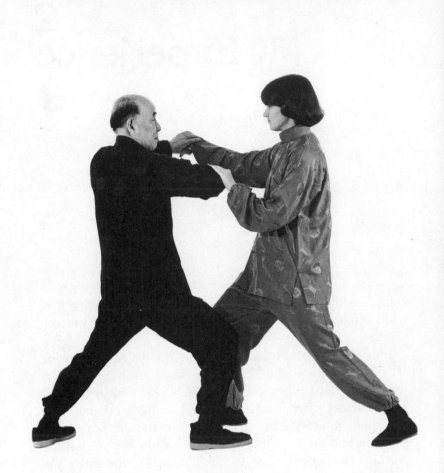

relaxation of body and mind lasting thirty minutes. For thirty minutes I really was in another world. It was an ideal world, peaceful and quiet. After the total relaxation of body and mind for this thirty minutes in the ideal world, I return to this one. This world so filled with tension, noise, politics, danger. It seems that half the population in the big cities has become crazed by it all. Have you ever tried to avoid these things? How?

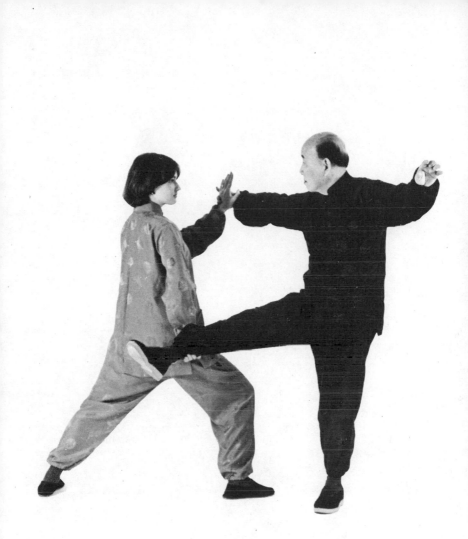

I have been teaching T'ai Chi in this country for more than a decade. The art has become more and more popular and I have many students including some Black Belt karate instructors who recently have begun to realize that the hard style is not enough and doesn't always work. If the opponent is stronger and faster, one is bound to lose to him. If one can master both hard and soft styles, one's techniques will reach the highest standard.

3
My Personal View

Man cannot live healthily without taking exercise. The *I Ching* [*The Book of Changes*] says: "As nature is always in motion, so should man act to strengthen himself without interruption." An ancient Chinese proverb says: "A door pivot will never be worm-eaten, and flowing water never becomes putrid." These aphorisms indicate that taking exercise leads to robust health. However, there are many kinds of exercise from which one will have to make a choice. Of all the exercises, I should say that T'ai Chi is the best. It can ward off disease, banish worry and tension, bring improved physical health and prolong life. It is a good hobby for your whole life, the older you are, the better. It is suitable for everyone—the weak, the sick, the aged, children, the disabled and blind. It is also an economical exercise. As long as one has three square feet of space, one can take a trip to paradise and stay there to enjoy life for thirty minutes without spending a single cent. So it is most advisable for us to adopt T'ai Chi.

From my more than thirty years experience of learning and practicing T'ai Chi, I formulated ten theorems for my daily guiding principles so I will know how to deal with people and myself:

1. Nobody can be perfect. Take what is good and discard what is bad.

2. If I believe entirely in books, better not read books. If I rely entirely on teachers, better not have teachers.

3. To remove a mountain is easy, but to change a man's temperament is more difficult.

4. If there is anything wrong with me, I don't blame others, I only blame myself.

5. If I want to live longer I must learn T'ai Chi and accomplish it both physically and mentally. To accomplish it mentally is much more difficult.

6. I must learn how to yield, to be tactful, not to be aggressive; to lose (small loss, small gain, great loss, great gain), not to take advantage of others; to give (the more one gives the more one will have).

7. Life begins at seventy. Everything is beautiful! Health is a matter of the utmost importance and all the rest is secondary. Now I must find out how to enjoy excellent health in my whole life and discover the way to immortality.

8. Make one thousand friends, but don't make one enemy.

9. One must practice what he preaches. Otherwise it is empty talk or a bounced check.

10. To conceal the faults of others and praise their good points is the best policy.

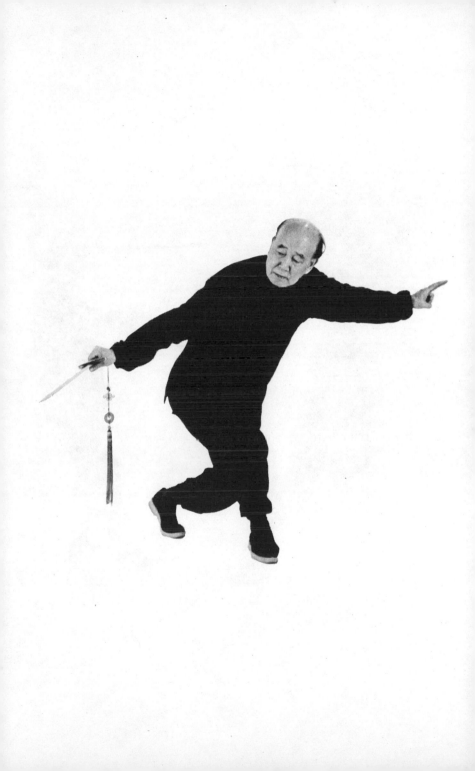

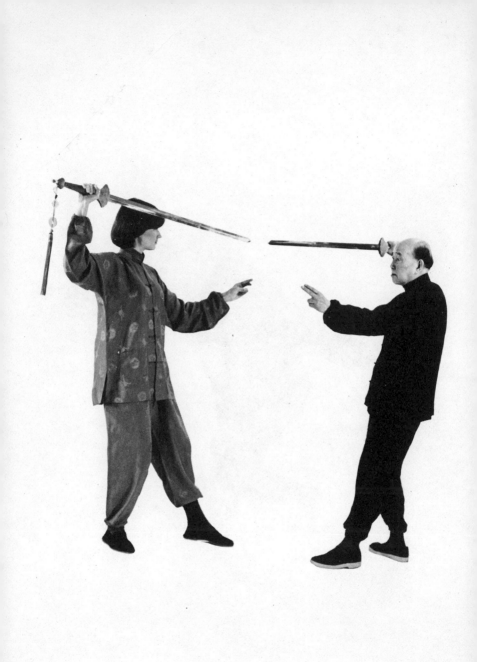

4
The Complete Set of T'ai Chi Exercises

The complete set of T'ai Chi exercises consists of:

1. T'ai Chi solo dance (right and left styles with 150 postures in each style)
2. Pushing Hands (active steps in fixed position, 8 movements)
3. Ta Lü (3 Ta Lü's, total of 26 postures)
4. T'ai Chi Dance with a partner (178 postures)
5. T'ai Chi Doubled-Edged Sword Dance (right and left styles, 60 postures in each)
6. T'ai Chi Sword Fencing (46 postures)
7. T'ai Chi Knife Dance (right and left styles, 32 postures in each)
8. T'ai Chi Knife Fencing (24 postures)
9. T'ai Chi Staff solo exercise (3 movements)
10. T'ai Chi Staff Fencing (8 postures)

All of the above can be practiced to music.

The Eight Trigrams

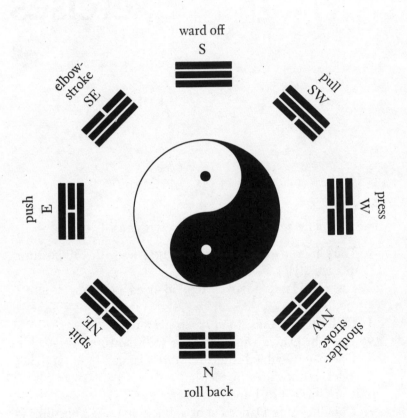

5
The T'ai Chi Classics

● T'ai Chi Ch'uan Classic
Chang San Feng, 13th Century
Translation and Commentary by T. T. Liang

In every movement the entire body should be light and agile and all of its parts connected like a string of pearls.

All of the postures must be practiced without the slightest constraint of energy and without any irrelevant tensions. Only then will the legs, arms, and trunk be weightless and nimble; only then will the body feel lively, alert, smooth, and free. The lightness is not an emptiness; it contains intrinsic energy. The agility is not superficial; it conceals a watchful awareness. Only when the entire body is light and agile in every movement can we talk about the second step, namely, that "all parts of the body must be connected like a string of pearls." This means that the movements must exhibit the incessant and continuous flow of a great river. If, similarly, our internal river (the blood-stream) circulates throughout the whole body without congestion, without hindrance, the body will become so alert and sensitized that an opponent will be at a loss to find even the slightest opening for attack. This T'ai Chi Ch'uan principle is of the utmost importance. But in order to reach the above-mentioned two stages, the following conditions must first be achieved:

1. Concentration of the mind
2. Complete relaxation of the body
3. Sinking of the ch'i to the tan t'ien and abiding by it so that breathing may be deep and slow.

A novice cannot be expected to acquire all of these conditions unless he is willing to apply himself to a long period of serious study and practice.

The ch'i should be stimulated and the spirit of vitality should be retained internally.

The ch'i is an inherent oxygen in the body for stamina and vitality. The ch'i of itself, latent in the body, is not sufficiently forceful to increase the flow of blood, but if the ch'i is persistently stimulated, it produces heat and becomes powerfully effective in activating the circulation of blood throughout the whole body without any discontinuity. The same principle is illustrated by the conversion of water into steam: the latent invisible power in water is made active enough, effective enough to drive the pistons of a powerful engine.

When the spirit of vitality is concentrated and retained internally, the heart (mind) will be tranquil and the entire body relaxed so that one may become alert and sensitive; disease can be prevented, and longevity enhanced. If, however, the spirit of vitality is diffused and exposed externally, there will be a widening of the eyes and increased body tension, resulting in circulatory congestion and loss of health. Moreover, since the desire of the mind is expressed by the spirit of vitality, your intentions will be readily apparent to an opponent who can then take the opportunity to attack you easily.

There should be neither deficiency nor excess, neither hollows nor projections, neither severance nor splice.

When one practices the postures, the whole body should be rounded out. The movements should not be uneven or irregular, suddenly high or suddenly low, but slow, smooth, even, effortless, and continuous so that the blood can circulate freely. The lowest vertebrae should not protrude; the entire spine should be plumb erect so that the spirit of vitality can reach to the top of the head. When stepping forward or backward, the body should be kept perfectly straight; inclination in any direction will disturb your balance (center of gravity) and will offer your opponent a "ready-to-be-beaten" posture.

The energy is rooted in the feet, develops in the legs, is directed by the waist, and moves up to the fingers. The feet, legs and waist must act as one so that when advancing and retreating you will obtain a good opportunity and a superior position.

During prolonged practice of the postures the intrinsic energy that is rooted in the soles of the feet (at the "Bubbling Well" point) develops to the legs, to the waist, to the spine, to the arms, to the fingers. When this energy has been fully liberated and distributed, the whole body will become activated and sensitized so that in stepping forward and backward you can obtain the "good opportunity" (i.e., you can detect the defects and susceptibilities of your opponent) and have the "superior position" (i.e., a faultless impregnable posture of your own that gives your opponent no opening for attack). This intrinsic energy is extraordinarily powerful if it is released from the spine with the whole body acting as one unit.

If you fail to gain these advantages, your body will be in a state of disorder and confusion. The only way to correct this fault is by adjusting your legs and waist.

The reason you cannot take advantage of the defect of your opponent and acquire a superior position of your own is because you adjust your position by using your hands rather than your legs and waist. The more you use the hands, the more clumsy and stiff your upper body will be. Consequently, your whole body will be in a state of disorder and confusion. Therefore, when you are in a disadvantageous position and cannot detect your opponent's defect, you must pay attention to the adjustment of your legs and waist. It has absolutely nothing to do with your hands, although you have hands.

The same principle applies to upward and downward, forward and backward, left and right. All the movements are to be directed by the consciousness within, rather than by the appearance without.

When you know how to adjust your waist and legs, your external action will follow your mental intent. But to know how to adjust your waist and legs is not an easy matter. You must first be conscious of your own plan, taking into consideration an accurate observation of your opponent in order to adapt yourself to the circumstances. In other words, you must have a clearly formulated idea of the goal and a perfected technique of achieving it before giving it outward expression. Therefore the movement of your waist and legs must be directed by a carefully mastered technique which is clear in your mind. Otherwise your movement will be simply a rash action or a "blindman's buff."

When attacking above you must not forget below; when striking to the left you must pay attention to the right; and when advancing you must have regard for retreating. If an attack is proposed upward, the initial intent must be downward. If you want to pull something upward, you must first push downward, causing the root to be severed and the object to be immediately toppled.

When engaging in combat you must adapt to all of the circumstances to create your own opportunities. When your opponent can see your attack only on one side and not on the other, he cannot detect the direction of your real attack. Since he cannot determine what your intention is, his body will be in a state of disorder and confusion and you will take this opportunity to knock him over. You must apply the "give-take" or "withdraw-attack" technique to uproot your opponent first, and then you can easily push him over.

The insubstantial and the substantial should be clearly discriminated. Each single part of the body has both a substantial and an insubstantial aspect at any given time and the body in its entirety also has an insubstantial and a substantial aspect. All the joints of the whole body are to be threaded together without the slightest severance.

When practicing T'ai Chi or when engaged in combat with an opponent, you must clearly differentiate the substantial and the insubstantial. You must be able immediately to change your substantial to insubstantial or vice versa, according to circumstances, so that he does not know you. But you know him perfectly well and thus you are second to none. When your opponent puts weight on your fingers, they become insubstantial and you immediately strike with your wrist. When he puts weight on your wrist, it becomes insubstantial and you immediately strike with your elbow. When he puts weight on your elbow, it becomes insubstantial and you immediately strike with your shoulder. When he puts weight on your shoulder, it becomes insubstantial and you immediately strike with your forehead. This is called "folding up technique." To illustrate by an example: when you knock the head of a long snake, its tail responds. When you knock its tail, its head responds. When you knock its back, its head and tail both respond.

Let me furnish another example: a man with great strength can lift an iron bar of one thousand pounds, but he cannot lift an iron chain of one hundred pounds because the latter is divided into many joints which are connected without severance so that no center of gravity can be traced. When practicing T'ai Chi or doing combat with an opponent you must employ the same principle.

T'ai Chi Ch'uan is also called Chang Ch'uan [Long Boxing] because its consecutive movements resemble the stream of a long river which rolls on ceaselessly. Ward Off, Roll Back,

Press, Push, Pull, Split, Elbow-Stroke, and Shoulder-Stroke in T'ai Chi Ch'uan are equivalent to Chien, Kun, K'an, Li, Hsun, Chen, Tui, *and* Ken *in the "Eight Trigrams." The first four postures represent the four cardinal points [i.e., South, North, West, and East]. The second four postures represent the four corners [i.e., Southwest, Northeast, Southeast, and Northwest]. The Five Attitudes—Advance, Retreat, Look to the Left, Gaze Right, and Central Equilibrium—in T'ai Chi Ch'uan are equivalent to the Five Elements of Chinese philosophy: Metal, Wood, Water, Fire, and Earth. Thus, the Eight Postures plus the Five Attitudes are generally termed the T'ai Chi Thirteen Postures.*

Note.—In many books, there is a footnote appended to this Classic which reads as follows: "This treatise has been handed down by Founder Chang San Feng of Wu Tang Mountain so that brave men everywhere can prolong their years and enhance longevity, not use the art merely as a means to martial skill."—*Ed.*

● The Mental Elucidation of the Thirteen Postures
Wang Chung Yueh of the Ming Dynasty
Translation and Commentary by T. T. Liang

Let the mind direct the ch'i so that it sinks deeply and steadily and can permeate the bones.

In practicing T'ai Chi the mind directs the ch'i which circulates through the entire body. The mind leads and the ch'i follows. All of the postures should be relaxed and firmly rooted. The mind should be tranquil and at rest. Then the ch'i can permeate the bones and become marrow. An internal intrinsic energy will be gradually developed which is tremendously powerful, strong, and limitless. Otherwise, the energy developed is only an external muscular force which is weak, ineffective, and limited.

Let the ch'i circulate throughout the entire body freely and without hindrance so that the body will follow the dictates of the mind.

If you want your ch'i to circulate freely through the whole body without hindrance, your postures must be even, effortless, harmonious, and comfortable. Then your hands, legs, and body will follow the dictates of the mind. If your postures are stiff and inactive, your ch'i cannot sink to the tan t'ien or circulate through the whole body; the body then will not follow the commands of your mind.

When you feel as if your head were suspended by a thread from above, your spirit of vitality will be raised and the defects of obtuseness and clumsiness will be no more.

The spirit of vitality is the essence of the whole body. No matter what you are doing, you will act rapidly and systematically with a full spirit of vitality. Without it your movements will be obtuse and clumsy. When practicing T'ai Chi, you must first raise your spirit of vitality To do this, your head must be upright and feel as if it were suspended in the air so that an active and alert energy will arise from the upper tan t'ien (a place between the two eyebrows) to the *pai hui* point (a place at the crown of the head). This is the correct way to raise your spirit of vitality when practicing T'ai Chi.

The mind and the ch'i must respond ingeniously and efficaciously to the exchange of substantial and insubstantial so as to develop an active and harmonious tendency.

When any part of your body contacts your opponent's body, you must change your substantial to insubstantial and vice versa in order to adapt to the circumstances. If you want to adapt to the circumstances in the nick of time, your mind and ch'i must respond ingeniously and efficaciously so as to develop an active and harmonious tendency. If your ch'i does not respond to the call of your mind and does not obey your commands, all your postures become inactive and clumsy and are called "ready-to-be-beaten" postures.

When attacking, the energy should be sunk deeply, completely relaxed, and concentrated in one direction.

You must find out: 1) the insubstantial part of your opponent's body, 2) the straight line of his body, and 3) his center of gravity. Then concentrate your energy in one direction and strike so that you can push him over far, far away. If these conditions are not met, the technique is of no use and is a mere blind strike.

When standing, the body should be erect and relaxed, able to sustain an attack from any direction.

When the head is upright and the vertebrae are erect, the body will not be inclined to the side. The mind should be open and at rest. Wait for the opponent's action in a cool and deliberate manner. The waist is like a perpendicular axletree and the hands and arms are like horizontal wheels, able to turn round at will to sustain attacks from any direction.

To direct the ch'i is like threading a pearl with nine crooked paths; there is no hollow which it does not penetrate.

A pearl with nine crooked paths has many winding hollows that the silken thread cannot penetrate. But an ant can carry the thread from one end of the pearl through all the openings to the other end. Similarly, the ch'i of itself cannot move very well. But the mind can direct it to circulate through the entire body without hindrance. If you know how to circulate your ch'i, you have already acquired this art and you are also on the way to immortality.

The energy when mobilized is like steel refined a hundred times over. There is no stiff adversary who cannot be overthrown.

The energy mobilized like steel refined a hundred times over is called intrinsic energy. It takes a long period of study and practice to attain it. When a piece of iron ore, after passing through a complicated process, has been refined into pure steel and is used to make swords and knives, they are so incomparably incisive that even iron can be scraped like mud. What about your opponent's body, made of flesh and blood? This is the meaning of the phrase, "No stiff adversary cannot be overthrown."

The appearance is like a hawk seizing a rabbit; the spiritual insight is like a cat catching a rat.

When attacking, your appearance is like a hawk seizing a rabbit. Usually a hawk wheels in the air in a leisurely and comfortable manner. As soon as it sees a rabbit below, it makes a rapid descent and suddenly attacks and seizes the rabbit, giving it no chance to defend itself and no time to take precautions. Your spiritual insight is like a cat catching a rat. When a cat is about to catch a rat, it shifts its weight to its hind legs and watches the rat with the full spirit of vitality in its eyes. If the rat does not move, the cat takes no action. When the rat, ready to escape, stirs ever so slightly, the cat moves quickly and catches the rat without fail.

In resting, be as still as a mountain peak; in moving, act like the current of a great river.

When you have practiced T'ai Chi for a long time, your feet will be firmly rooted like a mountain peak which cannot be removed by human strength. When you have mastered the techniques of all the postures, you can change from one posture to another, adapting to the circumstances so rapidly and swiftly that it resembles the current of a great river, giving the opponent no chance to resist.

To store up energy is like drawing a bow; to release energy is like shooting an arrow.

The intrinsic energy of T'ai Chi is concealed within rather than exposed without. In attacking, the intrinsic energy reserved within your body is as full as the energy of a bowstring, drawn to the fullest extent, ready to shoot. It is also like a rubber ball full of air. When your opponent touches your arm, it feels to him as soft as cotton, but he cannot press it down. During the moment of his astonishment and hesitation the arrow has already been shot without his notice. You are like a bow, and your opponent is like an arrow. Your attacking energy is so strong and fast that your opponent is cast out like an arrow shot from a bow.

Seek the straight from the curved; reserve energy before releasing it.

When your opponent attacks you, you must first withdraw your body and bend your arm to neutralize his attacking energy. Then store up your energy by inhaling, finding his body's straight line and center of gravity, and then immediately release your counterattacking energy by exhaling (a withdraw-attack technique).

The energy is released from the spine. The changing of steps must be in accordance with the movements of the body.

Before striking, hold in your chest, straighten your back, and concentrate your energy at the spine, waiting for the right moment to act. When striking, the energy is released from the spine so that you will obtain an intrinsic energy from the whole body acting as one unit. The body moves and the leg follows. Turn and change your body and steps according to circumstances, without fixed directions.

To withdraw is to attack; to attack is to withdraw. The energy is severed and again rejoined.

The movements of withdrawing and attacking cannot be separated. For instance, when your opponent strikes the left side of your body, you neutralize his striking energy by withdrawing and turning your body to the left and at the same time you strike him with your right hand. The striking force of your opponent's right hand is the same as the striking force from your right hand. It is similar to the action of a lever in physics. After attacking you must relax your whole body to be ready for the next action. When attacking, your energy is substantial (Yang) and when relaxing your whole body, it goes from substantial (Yang) back to insubstantial (Yin). When you strike, your energy becomes extreme Yang and the energy seems severed; when you relax your body, your energy is immediately connected by Yin.

When moving to and fro, "folding up" technique is to be applied; when advancing and retreating, it is necessary to turn the body and change the steps.

When your opponent strikes your hand, you withdraw it and immediately strike him with your wrist. When he strikes your wrist, you withdraw it and immediately strike him with your forearm (Ward Off posture). When he strikes your forearm, you withdraw it and immediately strike him with your elbow. When he strikes your elbow, you withdraw it and immediately strike him with your shoulder. When he strikes your shoulder, you withdraw it and immediately strike him with your forehead. This is called "folding up technique," and is also called the "variation of substantial and insubstantial." When your opponent strikes the left side of your body so fast that he gives you no chance to counterattack, you must yield and turn your body slightly to the left, while stepping back with your left foot in order to regain a favorable and superior position. After you have regained a superior position, you must turn your body slightly to the right if you want to counterattack with your left hand. If you step forward with your right foot, you must turn your body slightly to the left first and turn your body slightly to the right when striking with your left hand. This is the way of changing steps and turning the body.

From the most flexible and yielding you will arrive at the most inflexible and unyielding. If you can breathe correctly, your body will become active and alert.

When you practice T'ai Chi slowly, evenly, and effortlessly over a long period of time, an intrinsic energy will be developed, which is incredibly powerful and strong. Ordinarily, you breathe with your lungs (i.e., breathe from the upper chest alone). When you breathe in this manner, the ch'i remains ineffective. When you practice T'ai Chi and breathe with your abdomen, the abdominal respiration makes the ch'i that is latent in your body active and effective. The ch'i will then sink deeply into the tan t'ien from which it will circulate through the entire body without hindrance, so that your movements will be active and alert. This is beneficial for health and is also the way to immortality.

The ch'i should be cultivated naturally and harmoniously so as to avoid ill effects. The energy should be reserved slightly [by bending the limbs somewhat] so that there is a surplus in order to avoid exhaustion.

Mencius said, "I am skillful in cultivating my natural and magnanimous ch'i. Being nourished naturally and harmoniously, sustaining no injury, it fills up all between heaven and earth." To maintain firmness of will while doing no violence to the ch'i is the preliminary trial. Then calm your mind and breathe slowly and deeply without holding your breath. The mind directs the ch'i, which sinks deeply into the tan t'ien and then circulates through the whole body. This is what the *I Ching* means when it says, "Water and fire have been properly adjusted." Gradually the mind acts and the ch'i follows so that an internal energy is developed.

When you practice the postures, your arms and legs should be slightly bent and not be stretched to the fullest extent, so as to avoid tension. The curved line is like a river with many winding paths continuously flowing. When attacking, you should bend your arms slightly, so that after releasing energy you will still have a surplus in reserve. If you release your energy to the fullest extent without holding any back, your entire body will be tense and you will soon become exhausted. And if a stronger force immediately counterattacks you at this moment, you will be pushed over easily.

The mind is the commander; the ch'i is the flag; the waist is the banner.

When troops on the march are waging war, the commander gives the command, the military signal flag carries the command to the troops, and the big banner in front of the troops shows the directions. If the banner falls, all the troops will be dispersed and in disorder. It is the same when practicing T'ai Chi. The mind directing the ch'i is like the commander giving the command. The ch'i circulating through the whole body is like the military signal flag carrying the command to all the troops. The waist, which is the mainstay of the entire body's strength, is like a big banner indicating the direction while the troops march. The waist moves and the entire body follows. If the waist is broken off, the whole body will collapse.

At first seek open and expanded postures, later seek to make them close and compact so that a perfectly delicate and fine status will be attained.

When you practice T'ai Chi, at first your postures should be open and stretched out in order to loosen the muscles and circulate the blood so that your body will become stronger and stronger. Afterward, the postures should be made close and compact so that you can master all the techniques. When both physical well-being and functional use have been attained, you will finally have a delicate and fine status. From big circles you revert to small ones and from small ones you return to invisible ones—as it is said, "By enlarging they fill the universe; rolling up they can be concealed in a sleeve." When your movements have become invisible circles, you have mastered the function of T'ai Chi and fully entered into the profundities of this art.

If your opponent does not move, you do not move. At his slightest stir, you have already anticipated it and moved beforehand.

When joining hands with your opponent, you can strike him before he strikes because your hands are more sensitive and alert and can anticipate his slightest stir. Thus, you can strike him before he strikes you. That is to say, you know him very well, but he does not know you.

The energy appears relaxed and slackened but is in reality powerful and firmly rooted. The arms are ready to stretch, but not to the fullest extent. The energy may be broken off [i.e., discharged], but the mind-intent remains.

In striking, your energy appears soft and effortless, but internally it is powerful and strong. Your hands and arms are like steel bars wrapped with cotton. Your arms should not be stretched to the fullest extent; otherwise the entire body will be tense and your energy will be dispersed. After you have attacked, your energy is broken off, but your mind-intent remains so that you are still sensitive and alert, giving your opponent no chance to counterattack. As it is said, "The lotus root is broken off, but the fibers remain connected."

[It is also said] The mind is the leader and the body is the follower.

When you practice T'ai Chi, the mind is the active element, and the body is the passive. So the mind is of the first importance and the body is secondary. The body follows the mind as the shadow follows the substance. *Note.*—See another interpretation of this line in the commentary on the "Song of Pushing Hands."—*Ed.*

The abdomen is completely relaxed, enabling the ch'i to penetrate the bones; the spirit of vitality is at rest and the body is tranquil, permitting you to heed the intent of your mind.

When your abdomen is completely relaxed and sunk deeply without the slightest brute force, your breathing will be natural and harmonious. Your ch'i will rise and circulate throughout your entire body and eventually permeate your bones. When your spirit of vitality is at rest and your body is tranquil, you can heed the intent of your mind so that you can adapt to any circumstances without agitation and panic.

Always remember that once you act, everything moves, and once you stand still, all is tranquil.

When you move, your entire body must move systematically as one unit. Fragmentary and disorderly movements are to be avoided. When you stand still, your body and mind are both tranquil. The movements and resting places of arms, legs, hands, and body are synchronized. The phrase "In resting, be as still as a mountain peak; in action, be like the current of a great river" illustrates the same principle.

When you push and pull, withdraw and attack, your ch'i adheres to the back of your body and is gathered into the spine. Inwardly you strengthen your spirit of vitality; outwardly you appear peaceful and quiet.

When the ch'i adheres to the back of your body during the time of pulling and pushing, it will eventually permeate the bones, causing a natural intrinsic energy to be developed, which is tremendously powerful when released. Otherwise, only an external muscular force can be produced, which is weak and ineffective. When you strengthen your spirit of vitality inwardly, your ch'i will be concentrated. When you appear outwardly to be peaceful and quiet, you will maintain your equilibrium, your ch'i will be natural and harmonious, and your spirit of vitality will be tranquil so that your opponent cannot anticipate your action, and you give him no chance to take precautions. It is like a hawk seizing a rabbit. If you expose your spirit of vitality externally, your whole body will be tense and your opponent can detect your intentions easily.

Take steps like a cat walking; mobilize the energy as if reeling silk from a cocoon.

When practicing T'ai Chi, you most often step forward with your heel touching the ground first. The steps must be light and nimble so that the spirit of vitality will be concealed within. Mobilizing energy as if reeling silk from a cocoon signifies that the energy is active and alert, harmonious and even. If you jerk the thread while pulling, the silken strand will be broken, just as a jerk will cause the energy to be severed when practicing T'ai Chi.

If you pay full attention to your spirit of vitality and ignore your breathing, your striking force will be as strong as pure steel. If you pay attention only to your breathing, your blood circulation will be impeded and your striking force will be inactive and ineffective.

If you can cultivate your ch'i, an inherent "oxygen" of the Former Heaven, it will circulate from the tan t'ien through the entire body harmoniously, naturally, and evenly. When released, the resulting energy will be unlimited and tremendously powerful like pure steel. If you can only mobilize your breathing of the Latter Heaven, the ch'i will become clumsy and uneven, and blood circulation will be impeded so that the energy released will be weak, ineffective, and limited.

The ch'i is like a cartwheel; the waist is like an axletree.

The ch'i circulating through the whole body is like the turning of a cartwheel which is moving continuously, evenly, harmoniously, and actively. The waist, the controlling power of the whole body, is like an axletree which supports the entire wheel. All of the variations (of movement) are guided by the waist.

● T'ai Chi Ch'uan Treatise

Attributed to Wang Chung Yueh, Ming Dynasty
  Translation and Commentary by T. T. Liang

T'ai Chi (The Supreme Ultimate) springs from Wu Chi (The Limitless). It is the source of motion and tranquillity and the mother of Yin and Yang.

To stand still or motionless is called Wu Chi; to start moving is called T'ai Chi. Wu Chi creates T'ai Chi; T'ai Chi includes Yin (insubstantial) and yang (substantial). Yin and Yang transform themselves into all the manifestations of all things in the universe. So T'ai Chi is the mother of Yin and Yang.

In motion they separate; in tranquillity they fuse into one.

When you practice T'ai Chi, as soon as the mind has the intention of moving, the movement will be sent immediately to the whole body and the Yin and Yang will be developed and separated into two. When you stand still, the Yin and Yang will fuse into one and return to the original Wu Chi.

There should be no excess and no insufficiency. You bend as your opponent stretches out and expand as he contracts.

When you practice T'ai Chi or do combat with an opponent, there should be no excess and no insufficiency in your postures. No excess means that the body should be in perfect balance and equilibrium, neither inclining to the side nor leaning forward. If the opponent does not move, you do not move; when the opponent moves, you immediately respond. If your opponent finds any projections or hollows in your posture, it will be easy for him to take advantage of the opportunity and knock you over. Insufficiency means that while your opponent has already started to move, you do not know it and stay still and fall behind. Then you cannot discover your opponent's defects and there is no way to obtain a superior position of your own. So no excess and no insufficiency mean neither taking initiative nor falling behind, with no projections and no hollows. If you maintain a perfect equilibrium and your response is exactly correct and in the nick of time, you can act freely according to the nature of the changing situation.

To conquer the unyielding by yielding is termed "to withdraw"; to create a defective position in your opponent and obtain a superior position of your own is called "to adhere."

When your opponent strikes hard with his hand straight forward, you immediately withdraw your body and use the "Roll Back" posture to neutralize his striking force to the side of your body. This technique is called "to withdraw" (or dodge). When you have neutralized his striking force to the side, your opponent will be in a defective position. You immediately turn your body to the original position with your hand lightly touching his body. Now you are in a superior position and your opponent is in a defective position. This technique is called "to adhere."

You respond quickly to your opponent's fast action and slowly to his slow actions. Although the changes are numerous, the principle remains the same.

You should give yourself up completely, follow your opponent's action, and take no initiative of your own. If he attacks you fast, you must yield quickly; if he attacks you slowly, you can yield in a more leisurely manner. If he withdraws quickly, you must advance rapidly; if he retreats slowly, you can follow him up slowly so that you adhere closely and attach yourself to him without leaving any gap, like a sheet of medicated plaster stuck to his body. If you do this, and your hands and arms are completely relaxed without exerting the slightest external muscular force, they will be so sensitive and alert that they will adapt to circumstances in perfect coordination and harmony. If you put energy on your hands and arms, you can never give up yourself and follow others. No matter where your opponent turns or what kind of posture he uses against you, the principle of adherence mentioned above is the same.

From the mastery of all the postures you will apprehend "interpreting energy"; from apprehending interpreting energy, you will arrive at a complete mastery of your opponent without recourse to detecting his energy. But without a long period of arduous practice, you cannot find yourself suddenly possessed of a wide and far-reaching insight.

When practicing T'ai Chi, you must first learn all the postures correctly; then you should master all the postures by knowing their functional use; and finally you must know how to interpret energy. Interpreting energy means that you recognize whether your opponent's attack is fast or slow, long or short, real or unreal. At the opponent's slightest stir, you have already anticipated it and executed a counterattack before his attack reaches you. According to the *Art of War,* this is called, "dispatching troops after the enemy but arriving before he does." Nowadays beginners immediately want to know how to interpret energy and neglect the importance of practicing the postures. If one rejects the fundamentals and selects the incidentals, one can never reach the stage of interpreting energy. So if you want to arrive at a stage of divine transformation, you must first know how to interpret energy. If you want to know how to interpret energy, you must first master all the postures. Mastering all the postures results from constant practice. So in order to reach the height, one must begin from the bottom. The more you practice, the more you will become elegant and refined. And after exerting yourself for a long period of time, you will suddenly find yourself possessed of a wide and far-reaching insight. Then you will fully comprehend the body and function of T'ai Chi.

A light and nimble energy is to be preserved on the top of the head; the ch'i is to sink to the tan t'ien.

When you practice T'ai Chi, your whole body should be relaxed. When your whole body is completely relaxed, there should be a light and nimble energy preserved on the top of the head (the Pai Hui point). This energy is like a controlling power of your entire body to prevent you from falling or collapsing when your upper torso is completely relaxed. It is to be directed by the mind and is not to use external muscular force to push the head upward. When your head is held as if suspended by a thread from above, it will be perfectly erect, your mind will be tranquil and clear, and your whole body will feel light and nimble. Constant practice in this manner will brighten your eyes and ward off headaches. When the ch'i sinks to the tan t'ien and is directed by the mind, it will circulate through the entire body freely without hindrance. If the ch'i remains somewhere above the tan t'ien, it will hinder blood circulation and be detrimental to health.

There should be no inclination and no leaning. Suddenly disappear and suddenly appear.

No inclination means maintaining equilibrium of the body without inclining to the left or right side. If you incline to the left or right, you have already lost your balance, and it is easy for your opponent to push you over. No leaning means keeping your balance without leaning forward or backward. If you lean backward, it is very easy for your opponent to push you over when he suddenly steps forward and pushes you. If you lean forward when your opponent pushes you, you will immediately lose balance and if your opponent utilizes this opportunity to push you forward, you will be pushed over easily. This technique in T'ai Chi is called "withdraw and push." So in order to eliminate all of the above defects, you must stand with your body perfectly erect and completely relaxed, able to sustain an attack from any direction.

Suddenly disappear means to hide, your body immediately becoming insubstantial (Yin). Suddenly appear means to reveal yourself, your body immediately becoming substantial (Yang). When your opponent attacks, you withdraw your body which becomes insubstantial so that he is unable to put his energy onto your body. When he retreats, you immediately follow up to counterattack and your body immediately becomes substantial. So when you suddenly hide your body becomes Yin and when you suddenly reveal yourself your body becomes Yang. The opponent has no way to put energy onto your body and no place to escape and he is absolutely under your control.

When [the opponent] puts pressure on the left, the left becomes insubstantial; when pressure is brought on the right, the right becomes empty.

If the opponent attacks the left side of your body (i.e., puts a heavy pressure on your left side), you yield by withdrawing and turning your body to the left side so that your left side becomes insubstantial and the opponent's attacking force cannot find a solid resting place. If he strikes with his fist to the right side of your body, you yield by withdrawing and turning your body to the right so that his striking fist cannot find a target to hit. Your body is so light and nimble, so sensitive and alert that your opponent is unable to anticipate or comprehend you, and it is impossible for him to detect your empty and solid points. This is what is meant by "When the opponent puts pressure on the left, the left becomes insubstantial; when pressure is brought on the right, the right becomes empty."

Looking upward, it seems to become higher and higher; looking downward, it seems to become deeper and deeper.

If the opponent pushes you forward and upward by raising his body and hands, you should withdraw backward and upward by raising your body and hands. The higher he rises, the higher you follow, so it is impossible for him to reach you. If he presses you downward by squatting down, you also follow him, throwing yourself down and making him lose his balance. This is from the defensive point of view. When you raise your body and hands to push your opponent upward, he feels as if he is going to be thrown up to the sky. When you lower your body to push him downward, he feels that he is going to be knocked down into the earth. This is from the offensive point of view.

A long time ago on a summer day when T'ai Chi master Yang Pan Hou, the second son of the great master Yang Lu Ch'an, was cooling himself in the grain storehouse, a stranger suddenly appeared, asking the way to the residence of Yang Pan Hou. The Master answered, "I am Yang Pan Hou." The stranger immediately stretched out three fingers and pounced upon the Master. The Master withdrew his body slightly and, seeing a hut in the yard which was about eight feet high, beckoned to him saying, "Friend, please go up," and immediately knocked him up to the roof of the hut. Then he said, "Please hurry back home and find a doctor." The man escaped in great distress. A farmer who was on the spot asked the Master, "How could you knock him up to the roof of the hut?" The Master replied, "It is said in the T'ai Chi Classics, 'When one looks upward, it seems to become higher and higher.'"

A senior student who had studied from Master Yang for quite some time asked him to show a technique which was really good for practical use. The Master said, "All right, now I will throw you out in the shape of a silver ingot" (a large ingot weighing about fifty-three ounces, first cast under the Yüan Dynasty). The senior student laughed and said, "Please try and prove it." As soon as they began the match the senior student was immediately knocked down on the ground with his head and two feet facing the sky and his thighs touching the ground, exactly like the form of a silver ingot. The student's thighs were badly injured and it took him several months to recover after being treated by an herb doctor. So the senior often told the other students, " 'When one looks downward, it seems to become deeper and deeper,' describes a terribly fearful technique."

When advancing, one feels the distance incredibly long; when retreating, one feels it exasperatingly short.

When the opponent advances to attack you, you withdraw your body and induce him to come forward. Before his energy can reach your body, you use the technique of "Roll Back" to let his energy go to the side of your body. Then he can hit only the air and not your body. So he feels that the more he advances the longer the distance becomes. When he retreats, you immediately follow like a plaster adhering to his body, giving him no chance to escape. So he feels that the more he retreats the shorter the gap becomes.

A feather cannot be added to the body, nor can a fly alight.

When you have practiced T'ai Chi for a long period of time, your body becomes so sensitive and alert that as soon as you have the slightest contact with anything, you immediately feel it and sense how to respond to it. Even a weight as light as a feather you would not accept, but would try to neutralize. Your body is so light and nimble that even a fly cannot alight on it without setting it in motion. You can utilize the subtlety of your neutralizing energy to separate the legs of the fly and make it stumble as soon as it alights on your body. If you can do this, you have reached a high level in T'ai Chi.

One late summer's day master Yang Pan Hou was lying down to rest in the shade of the trees after practicing T'ai Chi. When the leaves dropped on his body, they all slipped off and fell to the ground so that not even one leaf remained. He frequently tested his achievement in T'ai Chi by lying on his bed, nipping a pinch of millet with his fingers, and putting it on his navel. With one exhalation all of the millet grains were shot out to the ceiling of the house like bullets shot from a gun. It is indeed very difficult to acquire a technique like that. One must exert oneself earnestly to reach it.

My opponent does not know me, but I know him quite well. If you can master all the techniques, you will become a peerless hero.

The opponent does not know me in any of the following respects: the substantial and insubstantial of my body, the straight line of my body, the long or short, swift or slow, real or fake of my strike, the high or low of my intention, my center

39

of gravity, or my superior or defective position. He cannot guess what kind of medicine I am carrying to sell in my gourd (a Chinese saying meaning a puzzling matter). But I know him quite well in all the ways mentioned above. I also know how to interpret his energy. My body is so sensitive and alert that at my opponent's slightest stir, I have already anticipated it and moved first, giving him no chance to take the offensive. It is said in the *Art of War*, "To know your own plans and be acquainted with those of the enemy is the sure way to victory." So to master all the techniques is the way to become a peerless hero in T'ai Chi.

In martial arts there are many other schools. Although they differ in postures, they do not go beyond reliance on the strong defeating the weak, the swift conquering the slow, or the slow yielding to the quick and the weak being defeated by the strong. But these are all the result of innate physical endowments and do not relate to techniques acquired by study and experience.

In the martial arts there are many schools. Most of them emphasize the strong defeating the weak and the swift conquering the slow. Clearly, they all rely on external muscular force to win. This is not the way of T'ai Chi. The art of T'ai Chi is entirely different. To give up oneself and follow others, to discriminate clearly between the substantial and insubstantial, to relax the entire body and sink the ch'i to the tan t'ien, to conquer the most unyielding with the most supple and yielding, to use intrinsic energy and not external muscular brute force, to deflect the momentum of one thousand pounds with a trigger force of four ounces—these are the fundamental techniques of T'ai Chi. This is the orthodox teaching of the art. So any martial art that relies on the strong to defeat the weak or the swift to conquer the slow may not be mentioned with T'ai Chi as an art of self-defense.

If one examines the principle of deflecting a momentum of a thousand pounds with a trigger force of four ounces, clearly it is not brute force that wins.

When one has mastered the art of T'ai Chi, the body is so sensitive and alert that one can easily neutralize an attacking force of a thousand pounds with the technique of "Roll Back," so the attacking force will be neutralized to the side of one's body. Then, by applying a mere four ounces of push-and-pull energy, one finds the opponent's defect, obtains a superior position of one's own, and knocks the opponent over.

If one sees an old man defending himself and defeating a great number of men, what has this to do with swiftness?

"Old man" can refer to a man eighty or ninety years of age. When an old man like this can defend himself and defeat a great number of men, it indicates that the old man has been practicing T'ai Chi and has acquired all its techniques. Through the practice of T'ai Chi the old man's sinews, tendons, and bones become stronger and stronger. The older he gets, the more vigorous he becomes. He can enjoy good health his whole life through. In the phrase, "What has this to do with swiftness?" the word "swiftness" means mere speed, confused and disorderly, which can be of no value for practical use. Swiftness with perfect technique is real swiftness which can be put to practical use.

Stand like a balanced scale; move actively like a cartwheel.

"Stand like a balanced scale" means that the body should be erect and relaxed without inclining or leaning in any direction, able to withstand attacks from all directions. "Move actively like a cartwheel" means that the lowest vertebrae are plumb erect and the head is straight as if suspended from above, so that a perpendicular line is formed like the axis of a cartwheel. Then in any movement the turning of the body is active like the turning of a wheel. The T'ai Chi Classics say: "When the opponent puts pressure on the left, the left becomes insubstantial; when pressure is brought on the right, the right becomes empty." Neutralize also means attack. Your body is so light and nimble that it turns like a cartwheel and all the attacking

41

energy from an opponent is neutralized to the side of your body.

If you keep your weight on one side you can adapt to all circumstances; if you "double-weight," your actions will be impeded.

When riding a bicycle, if you step on the pedal with your right foot, putting weight on it while leaving the left foot unweighted, the wheel of the bicycle can turn and move forward without hindrance. If you step on the pedals trying to put weight on both feet at the same time, the wheel will be impeded and will not turn at all. The principle of T'ai Chi is the same. When you are ready to push an opponent with two hands attached to his body, you must find the substantial and insubstantial part of his body first and then push with one hand, using no energy with the other hand. Then he will be pushed over easily. If you push him using energy with both hands, you are in danger of losing balance and being pushed over if he uses "Roll Back" and suddenly turns his body to the side.

If you step forward with your right foot, you must first shift your weight entirely to the left foot so that the movement will be light and nimble. When you practice the solo postures of T'ai Chi, if you step forward with your right foot your right heel must touch the ground first, as you shift all your weight to the left foot, leaving no weight on the right foot. As soon as you find that the place you are touching with the right heel is solid and secure, you shift your weight to the right foot. If you find that the place is not solid or is insecure, you can immediately withdraw your foot to the rear. If you step forward with weight on both feet, you will immediately fall into a trap. If you step recklessly in daily life, you may be hurt or become involved in a fatal accident. Furthermore, if you step forward with weight on both feet, the opponent can sweep your foot and you will be easily knocked over. This is why you can adapt to any circumstance by keeping your weight on one side. And if you double-weight, your actions will be impeded, so from the

T'ai Chi point of view you will be in a "ready to be beaten posture."

We often see one who has painstakingly practiced T'ai Chi for several years but cannot neutralize an attacking energy and is generally subdued by an opponent. This is because he has still not understood the fault of double-weighting.

To collide with your opponent, to push your opponent with energy on both hands, to put energy in your upper torso when doing the postures, to step forward and backward with weight on both feet, and to find the opponent's defect and obtain a superior position of your own by using a hand block are all defects of double-weighting. These defects must be avoided. Otherwise even a whole lifetime of practice will be of no avail. It will be of no use for self-defense or as a physical exercise.

If you want to avoid this defect, you must know Yin and Yang.

If you want to avoid the defect of double-weighting you must know the principle of Yin and Yang. Yin is insubstantial and Yang is substantial. When the opponent attacks the left side of your body, you must withdraw your body and shift your weight to the rear foot, neutralizing the attacking energy by turning your body to the left. The left then becomes insubstantial while you counterattack with your right hand, which becomes substantial.

To adhere is to withdraw; to withdraw is to adhere. Yang does not leave Yin and Yin does not leave Yang. The coordination of Yin and Yang can be called interpreting energy.

When your opponent strikes you (i.e., a substantial or Yang force comes to your body), you should neutralize his striking energy by yielding and withdrawing so that your body becomes insubstantial or Yin. Your hands or another part of your body should adhere to his body without leaving any gap. When your opponent withdraws his body (which then becomes insubstantial or Yin), you should immediately follow up, letting your hands lightly adhere to his body leaving no gap, so that you are ready to attack at any moment with Yang. By moving back and forth in this way, the Yin and Yang mutually wax and wane. This is called, "Yin does not leave Yang; Yang does not leave Yin." If you can adapt yourself to the circumstances without the slightest error, the Yin and Yang will be in perfect coordination and you will have acquired the technique of interpreting energy in T'ai Chi Ch'uan.

After you have learned to interpret energy, the more you practice, the better your skill will be, and by examining thoroughly and remembering silently, you will gradually reach a stage of total reliance on the mind.

After you have practiced the postures, Pushing Hands, Ta Lü, and the T'ai Chi Dance for a long period of time, you will reach the stage of interpreting energy. Then the more you practice the more refined and delicate your skill will be. And you can increase your skill still further by continuously remembering in silence and examining thoroughly what you have learned from teachers and books. Gradually your skill will reach such a high level that your body will immediately respond to the dictates of your mind.

The fundamental point is to forget oneself and follow others. But most people misunderstand it and sacrifice the near for the distant.

When you engage an opponent in combat, you must follow his movements and take no initiative of your own. Old Master Yang Ch'eng Fu often said, "If you follow others, your body will be light and nimble but if you take initiative, your whole body will be clumsy and confused." The T'ai Chi Classics say, "If your opponent does not move, you do not move. At his slightest stir, you have already anticipated it and moved beforehand." "His slightest stir . . ." means that your opponent is already moving so that you can find his defects and take this opportunity to attack. This is the accurate and correct technique. If you take initiative of your own, you must move your hands and feet up and down, back and forth in a state of confusion, looking for the opponent's defects in order to attack. If you do this, it will be easy for the opponent to detect your defects and knock you over. So this is an inaccurate and incorrect way. Now let me cite an example to illustrate the point. When a cat sees a mouse in the distance and is ready to catch it, the mouse does not move. The cat does not move either but watches, appearing peaceful and quiet outwardly, but inwardly alert and ready to attack at any moment. When the mouse, ready to escape with its life, makes the slightest stir, the cat springs upon it, catches, and holds the mouse in its mouth. I have often seen this when I was young; the cat never missed even once. When the mouse's body stirs ever so slightly, the cat has already anticipated it and knows where the mouse is going to escape. It then runs in a short-cut way and intercepts the mouse. In the *Art of War* this is called, "Dispatching troops later, but arriving first (through a short-cut)." It is a different story when a dog tries to catch a squirrel. As soon as it sees a squirrel, the dog looks very nervous and tense and begins to bark, giving the squirrel plenty of warning. The dog then immediately runs to the squirrel, not noticing whether the squirrel is moving or not. As soon as the dog reaches the spot, the squirrel has already escaped. The dog, dumfounded on seeing that the squirrel has disappeared, gives a few more barks, and wonders why it could not catch the squirrel. The squirrel looks down from high in the tree and seems to chide the dog, "Don't bother me next time, you can never catch me." I have seen this many times in a park in New York City and the dog has never once caught the squirrel.

This is what is called, "a slightest error or deviation will result in wide divergence (from the true way)." Therefore the student cannot but thoroughly discriminate the right and wrong. For this reason the Classics have been made.

The principles and theories of T'ai Chi are so profound and abstruse and the applications are so subtle and ingenious that you must find out the absolutely accurate and correct way to learn and practice. If what you have learned is not quite correct and accurate, the minimal error will keep you handicapped and you will fall behind by a thousand miles. You will also lose the functional use of T'ai Chi. Students must heed this well.

● Song of the Substance and Function of the Thirteen Postures

The thirteen basic postures must never be regarded lightly. The original source of their meaning is in the waist.

Originally there were only thirteen postures in T'ai Chi Ch'uan. Through progressive changes the entire series has now evolved to one hundred and fifty postures. The thirteen postures of T'ai Chi possess the potential of prolonging life and the art of resisting insult. The theories and principles are so profound and abstruse that it is very difficult to acquire this art. The words "must never be regarded lightly" contain a measure of advice and an earnest hope that the Thirteen Postures which are so important to human life must not be regarded as negligible.

The waist is the mainstay of all the T'ai Chi movements, so it is called "the axletree of the wheel." It is far more important than other parts of the body because it has the function of strengthening the heart and circulating the blood in the vessels. The four limbs rely on it to revolve and the whole body depends on it for support. This is why the principle of "the original source of their meaning is in the waist" has been developed.

In changing and turning from substantial (Yang) to insubstantial (Yin) and vice versa, one must pay close attention; ch'i will circulate throughout the entire body without the slightest hindrance.

The movements of changing and turning from substantial to insubstantial and vice versa contain elements of expanding and contracting, opening and closing, revolving, advancing and retreating. When practicing the postures, one must pay close attention to all the movements, doing them lightly, vividly, effectively, comfortably, and harmoniously. All must be directed by the mind so the ch'i will circulate through the entire body without the slightest hindrance. If the movements are propelled by external muscular (brute) force, the whole body will be tense, the ch'i will be impeded, and the free circulation of ch'i and blood will be stopped.

Inwardly tranquil, one responds to a forceful action while maintaining an unruffled attitude. Manifest your inscrutable techniques to accord with an opponent's changing actions.

Tranquillity and action are two extremely contradictory instincts. In the literal sense tranquillity means to guard or protect and action means to attack. ("Literal," that is, as a T'ai Chi technical expression.) While motionless, be as still as a mountain peak, maintaining a firmly rooted posture without floating. When moving, act like the current of a great river, rolling on ceaselessly to meet each changing condition. Ordinarily a person maintains a quiet attitude. But when one part of the body receives a stimulus, that part will move and the rest of the body will immediately follow. The internal organs (the viscera), however, should remain tranquil so that one can meet the arising circumstances with an easy manner. Otherwise the entire body will be scattered and confused, making it impossible to detect the defects of an opponent or to maintain one's own superior position. "The mind and ch'i must respond ingeniously and efficaciously to the exchange of substantial and insubstantial so as to develop an active and harmonious tendency . . . the entire body is so light and sensitive that a feather will be felt and so pliable that a fly cannot alight on it without setting it in motion. Your opponent cannot fathom your moves, but you can anticipate his quite well." If one can

47

manifest all these inscrutable techniques to accord with the opponent's changing actions, one can be assured of winning the bout. But one cannot reach such a high level without hard study and diligent practice over a long period of time.

Pay special attention to your every posture and seek out its hidden meaning, then you can acquire this art without exerting excessive effort.

In every posture one should know his own variations of substantial and insubstantial and how to turn his body and vary his steps when advancing and retreating. At the same time one must also concentrate the mind, relax the body, and sink ch'i to the tan t'ien in order to estimate and take cognizance of the opponent's intent and substantial and insubstantial aspects. In this way one can make an effective counterattack; the hands will be able to do what the mind wishes without wasting time and effort.

Pay attention to your waist at all times. When the abdomen is completely relaxed, the ch'i will soar up (and circulate through the entire body).

Here it again reminds the student to pay attention to the waist. When the abdomen is relaxed, the mind will be at ease and the ch'i will sink to the tan t'ien and circulate throughout the entire body without impediment. The body will feel light and nimble. In times of practical application, you will act as effectively as you desire.

When the lowest vertebrae are plumb erect, the spirit of vitality reaches to the top of the head. When the top of the head is held as if suspended from above, the whole body feels light and agile.

There is a direct connection between the spine and the coccyx. It is an important passage for the rise and fall of the ch'i. When the lowest vertebrae are erect, forming a straight line with the occiput, the spirit of vitality will rise to the top of the head and the mind will be clear and alert. When the head is upright and the top of the head held erect as if suspended from above, the whole body will maintain a perfect balance and feel light and nimble. When a man stands, the top of his head points to heaven and his feet join the earth, forming a perpendicular line. His mind is clear and alert. Other animals like the lion, tiger, horse, and ox are different. When they stand their heads and spines are in a horizontal line. Their bodies are strong, but their minds are dull and stupid. That is why human beings are the cleverest creatures in the world.

Examine and investigate carefully and thoroughly. Whether bending, stretching, opening, or closing, let it take its natural way.

Examine carefully the theories and principles of the Thirteen Postures and investigate the functional use of how to neutralize, grasp, and change from substantial to insubstantial. Bending (contracting inward) is to mobilize the energy like drawing a bow, and stretching is to issue the energy like shooting an arrow. Opening is stretching out the hands, arms, and legs, turning the body and limbs in a light and lively manner. Closing is adhering closely to an opponent and then issuing energy. (Note: one must adhere to the opponent first, then issue energy.) As the "Song of Pushing Hands" says, "Entice him to advance; when his energy is emptied, adhere to him (closing) and issue energy." When you have acquired all the techniques implied in the movements you will be able to apply them freely without exerting much effort.

To enter the gate and be guided onto the correct path one requires verbal instruction from a competent master. If one practices constantly and studies carefully, one's skill will take care of itself.

If one wants to know the essentials of this art one must have a good teacher who can explain all the correct theories and principles and demonstrate the practical use of each technique. The teacher, however, can only lead the student to the correct gate, he cannot compel him to go further. Somewhere inside the gates masses of gold and diamonds lie hidden. It is up to the student to go beyond the door and into the inner rooms to search for the treasure. So in order to acquire the art one must have a determined and enduring mind, ready to persevere and study hard. If one relies entirely on the teacher one will never find the treasure. So we have an old saying, "If you believe entirely in books, better not read books; if you rely entirely on teachers, better not have teachers."

If one asks about the correct standard of substance and function, [the answer is that] the mind and ch'i direct, and the flesh and bones follow.

If one asks, "What is the correct method of learning T'ai Chi?" the answer is that the mind and ch'i are the master and the flesh and bones are the assistants. If one wishes to reach the highest level of this art, one must first place emphasis on the cultivation of the mind and ch'i internally. Strengthening external muscular capabilities is secondary.

Carefully examine what the ultimate purpose is—the enhancement of longevity, rejuvenation, and immortality.

If one asks, "What is the purpose of learning the Thirteen Postures of T'ai Chi?" the answer is that the object of prime importance is to keep good health and increase one's resistance (to diseases, tensions, etc.) so as to live longer and find the way to immortality (i.e., follow the Taoist doctrines). In comparison with this, the practical skills of this art are trifles.

The Song of the T'ai Chi Thirteen Postures contains 140 Chinese words. Each one is genuine and true doctrine which explains fully and without reservation the meaning and purpose of T'ai Chi. If you do not seek carefully in the direction indicated above, your time and effort will be spent in vain and you will have cause to sigh with regret.

In conclusion it stresses again the genuineness of each word of explanation which present the only correct way to acquire this art physically and mentally. If the student does not study with diligence and examine carefully according to what the Song indicates, his time and effort will all be in vain.

6
The Essentials of T'ai Chi Ch'uan

1. The theories behind T'ai Chi Ch'uan (often simply called "T'ai Chi") are not easy to comprehend because of their depth and subtlety. The techniques, moreover, are quite difficult to acquire.

2. Correct method is of the utmost importance. One must learn things in proper sequence and allow progress to come in a gradual and natural manner. Otherwise an entire lifetime of study will be to no avail.

3. The T'ai Chi Ch'uan Classic states, "The movement of upward and downward, backward and forward, left and right are to be directed by the mind-intent and not by external muscular force."

4. The mind-intent refers to the internal spiritual function and the outer aspect refers to the movements of the postures motivated by external muscular force.

5. If every movement can be directed by the mind-intent within and manifested without, then the internal spiritual

aspect and external physical aspect will be united. Upper and lower parts of the body will move in unison. Thus the body will instantly follow the dictates of the mind and the ch'i, and intrinsic energy will immediately reach the intended point.

6. In the "Song of the Thirteen Postures" it is said, "Pay special attention to your every posture and seek out its hidden meaning, then you can acquire this art without exerting excessive effort."

7. It is evident that if from the beginning you try to use mind-intent to direct the movements, your skill will be improved by leaps and bounds; gradually when you have mastered the use of your mind you will be able to acquire all the techniques. Therefore the most important guiding point of T'ai Chi Ch'uan is the use of mind-intent to direct the movements.

8. If one can grasp this important guiding point and constantly comprehend the principles, one will obtain the very essence of T'ai Chi. As the T'ai Chi Classics say, "The more you practice, the more you will master the art. By silently remembering and thoroughly comprehending you will eventually reach a state of complete reliance on the mind . . ."

9. T'ai Chi Ch'uan is a combination of civil and martial aspects. The civil aspect stresses principles and the martial aspect stresses techniques. Both aspects must be taken into account; neglecting either one is not a real T'ai Chi Ch'uan.

10. The civil aspect is called Tao (principle) and the martial aspect is called skill (technique). In the real T'ai Chi Ch'uan the civil and martial aspects are equally important.

11. Tao emphasizes internal cultivation; skill emphasizes external discipline. Cultivating one's nature (temperament) is

called internal development; training the muscles and bones is called external development. The internal cultivation of temperament and the external training of muscles and bones are both important; neither can be lacking. So we can see that the unification of both civil and martial aspects, the equal importance of Tao and techniques, and the internal cultivation with external training are the very best methods for beginners to learn T'ai Chi.

12. When one practices T'ai Chi, one must direct all the movements by mind-intent. As the "Song of the True Interpretation of T'ai Chi" says, "Formless and imageless (forgetting oneself), the whole body completely relaxed (internal and external united into one), and forgetful of everything returning to the natural way (following the desire of the mind) . . ." This indicates that mind-intent has reached the ultimate stage.

13. There are three important T'ai Chi Classics. The first, called the T'ai Chi Ch'uan Classic, was created and handed down by Chang San Feng, a Taoist of the late Sung Dynasty. This classic begins by saying, "In every movement the entire body should be light and agile and all of its parts connected like a string of pearls." The opposite of light and agile is heavy and clumsy and the opposite of connected like a string of pearls is dispersed and confused. This indicates the coordination of substantial and insubstantial and discloses the objective of the fundamental principle of T'ai Chi.

14. It goes on to say, "The ch'i should be stimulated and the spirit of vitality should be concealed within." This again emphasizes the importance of the internal cultivation of ch'i and the spirit of vitality.

15. The Classic continues, "There should be no deficiency and no excess, no hollows, no projections, no severance and no splice." These defects result from using external muscular

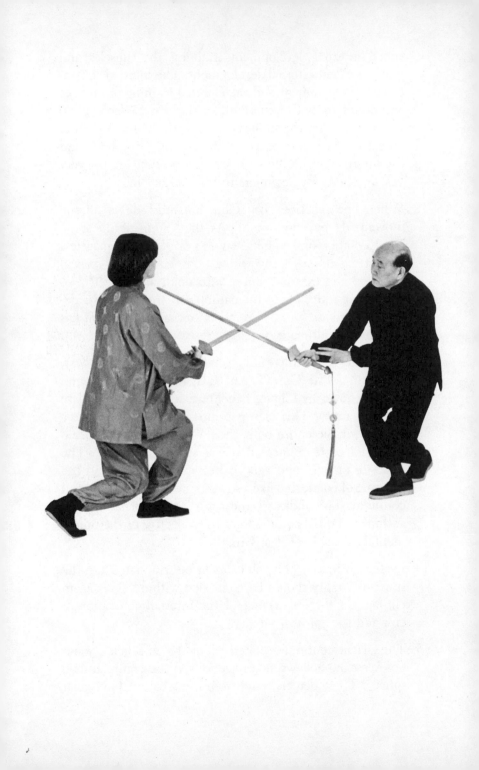

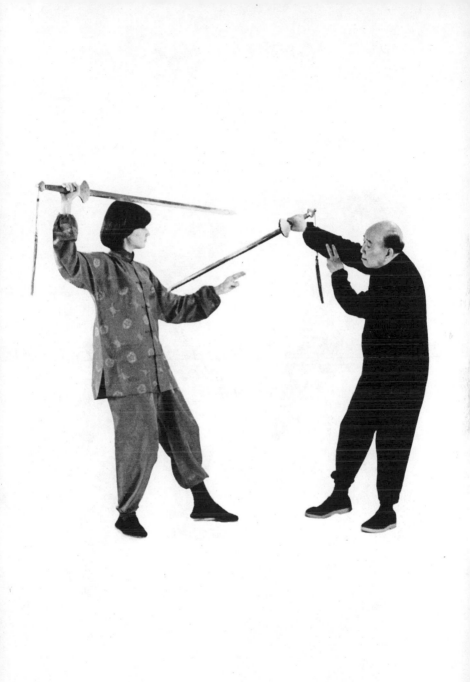

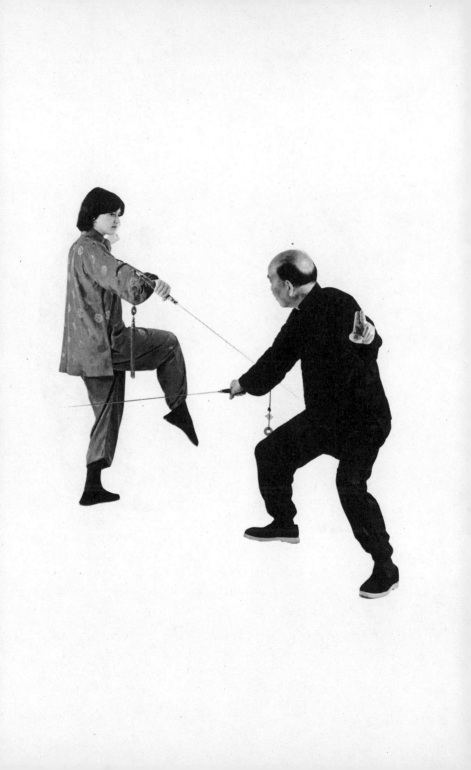

force. If, however, the mind-intent is employed to direct the movements of the body, the entire body will be relaxed and pliable so as to fulfill the requirement of being "light and agile, its parts connected like a string of pearls."

16. And again it says, "The energy is rooted in the feet, develops in the legs, is directed by the waist, and moves up to the fingers. The feet, legs, and waist must act as one so that when advancing and retreating you will obtain a good opportunity and a superior position." The above explains the systematic method of practice.

17. The three paragraphs above have revealed the important points of the principles, methods, and functions. The principles indicate the reason why; the methods indicate what ought to be; and the functions reveal the efficacy of both the principles and the methods. These three are all interdependent and mutually support each other in practice. Not one of them should be lacking. By practicing in this way, one will be in accord with what is called, "the unification of civil and martial aspects, the equal importance of principle and technique, and the combined cultivation of internal and external."

18. The second important treatise was written by Wang Chung-yueh of the Ming Dynasty. In the beginning it says, "T'ai Chi (The Supreme Ultimate) is evolved from Wu Chi (Infinity) and is the mother of Yin and Yang. In movement the two become separated, in stillness they combine into one. There should be no excess and no insufficiency. You yield as the opponent stretches out." The above indicates that T'ai Chi is derived from the principles of the *I Ching*.

19. The treatise then says, "To conquer the strong by yielding is called withdrawal; to make a favorable position of your own and a defect in your opponent is termed adherance. You respond quickly to fast action and respond to slow

action in a leisurely manner. Although the changes are numerous, the principle is the same (that of an all-pervading unity)." The above includes all the principles and techniques of T'ai Chi.

20. The third treatise is Wang Chung-yueh's "Mental Elucidation of the Thirteen Postures." It emphasizes especially the methods of practice with the utmost delicacy and accuracy.

21. In the beginning this treatise states, "Let the mind direct the ch'i . . ." "Mind" refers to mind-intent, which is a human perception. This is the leading principle of the entire treatise.

22. It goes on to say, "The mind is the commander, the ch'i is the flag, and the waist is the banner." And further—"The mind leads and the body follows . . ." When performing all of the movements, one's mind-intent is directed to the spirit of vitality and not to external use of breath or physical force." These phrases all indicate the importance of mind-intent when practicing T'ai Chi.

23. The above three treatises include all the essential aspects of T'ai Chi Ch'uan. Students must make a thorough investigation and have a deep understanding in order to acquire this art.

7
The Ten Guiding Points of T'ai Chi Ch'uan

1. Relax.

The word *sung* is usually translated into English as "relax." The basic meaning of the word relax is to become looser or less firm in the muscles, to become less tense or stern in one's features, or to give up one's energy. From the T'ai Chi point of view, however, the word relax can represent only a part of the meaning of the Chinese *sung*. Since I cannot find an equivalent in English to express fully the meaning of *sung*, I must use the word relax, which is about the closest word to it. The principle of *sung* implies loosening one's muscles and releasing one's tensions, giving up one's energy externally but preserving it internally so that one's body will be sensitive and alert enough to adapt itself to any circumstance. Otherwise, it will be merely a body collapse, which has no ability to meet an emergency.

2. Sink.

To sink means to relax completely. The whole body (the upper torso, the waist, the thighs and legs) should all be relaxed. All the energy should be concentrated in the "Bubbling Well

Point," a hollow place in the middle of the sole of the foot. When one has reached this high level of development, the ch'i will sink deeply to the tan t'ien, and one's movements will be light and nimble. The body will be so sensitive and alert that it can feel the weight of a feather, and a fly would not be able to alight on it without setting it in motion.

3. The chest should be held in, the back straightened, the shoulders sunk, and the elbows lowered.

When the chest is slightly held in, the ch'i will sink to the tan t'ien and the blood will circulate throughout the whole body without hindrance. Otherwise, the ch'i will come up and accumulate in the chest, causing the top of the body to be heavy and the bottom light, and the feet to be easily uprooted.

When the back is straightened, the energy will be collected in the spine so that the whole body will act as one unit and the energy that is issued will be tremendously powerful. Otherwise the energy will be dispersed.

The shoulders should be sunk, so the ch'i will sink to the tan t'ien. If the shoulders are shrugged, ch'i will immediately rise up to the chest, and the entire body will be heavy and clumsy so that the application of energy will be to no avail.

The elbows should also be lowered. The elbows and shoulders are closely connected. If the elbows are raised, the shoulders will be immediately affected.

4. A light and nimble energy should be preserved on the top of the head. The lowest vertebrae should be erect.

The head should be straight and the whole body should be completely relaxed without exerting the slightest external force. Keep a light and nimble energy on the top of the head as if you were suspended from above to prevent you from collapsing. The lowest bertebrae should be erect so that the mind will be clear. When the top of the head feels as if it were suspended from above, the whole body feels light and nimble. Human beings are the cleverest creatures in the world because their heads reach to heaven and their feet stand on the earth.

5. All the movements are directed by the mind. One does not use external muscular force.

It is said in the Classics: "Use the mind to direct the movements, which will then be light and agile. If you use external muscular force to direct the movements, they will be heavy and clumsy." When one practices T'ai Chi, the whole body should be completely relaxed, not exerting the slightest clumsy force in the muscles, bones, or blood vessels. If one does not restrain oneself (by using clumsy muscular force), one's movements will be light and nimble, and the body can be turned at will. There are some who doubt this and say, "If you don't use energy, how can you develop energy?" The answer is that we have sinews and (blood) vessels in our body which are like underground water courses. The water will flow continuously when the courses are not blocked, just as the ch'i will circulate through the whole body when the sinews and vessels are not obstructed. If the sinews and vessels are filled with clumsy energy, the ch'i flow and blood circulation will be impeded, the turning of the body will not be light and agile, and even the slightest stir of any part of the body will be shaky and tottering.

If you use the mind instead of muscular force to direct your movements, then the ch'i will follow where mind-intent directs. So day by day the ch'i and blood will circulate through the whole body without hindrance. If one practices in this manner for a long period of time, one will acquire the real intrinsic energy. In the T'ai Chi Classics it is said: "From the most flexible and yielding one will arrive at the most powerful and unyielding." When one has mastered the techniques of T'ai Chi, one's arms are like iron bars wrapped in cotton, and the weight of both arms is tremendously heavy.

6. Upper parts and lower parts follow each other, and the body acts as one unit.

When the hands move, the body and legs immediately move also so that the whole body acts simultaneously. As it says in the T'ai Chi Classics: "It is rooted in the feet, develops in the legs, is directed by the waist, and functions through the fingers.

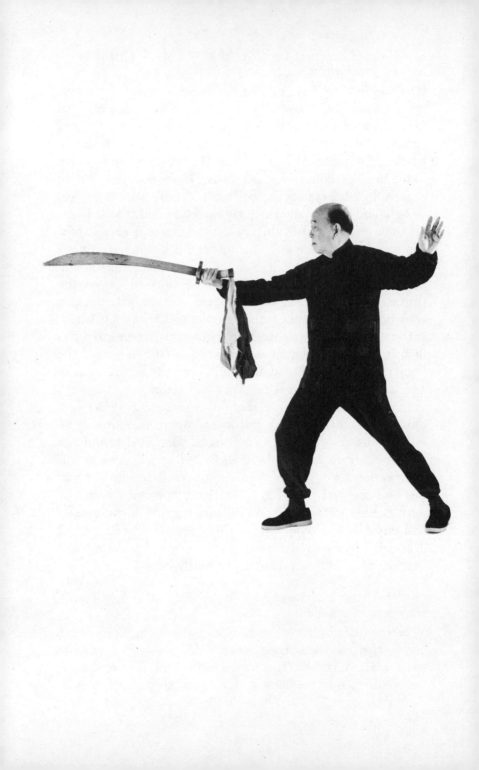

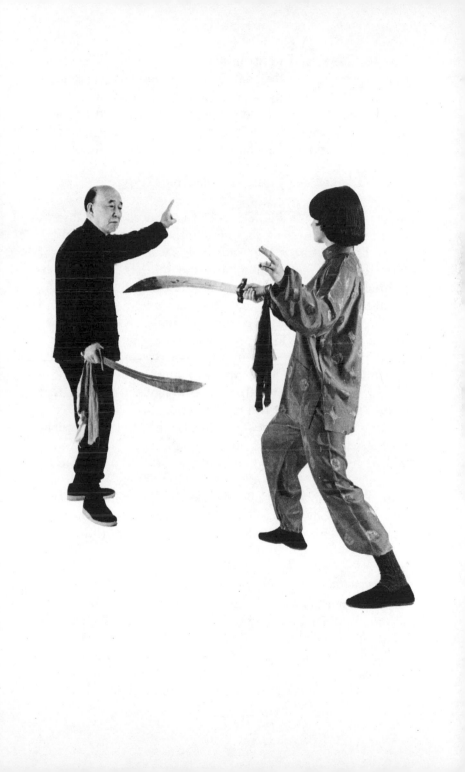

The feet, legs, and waist must act as one unit. When one moves, every part of the body is moving, and when one stops, every part of the body is tranquil so that in advancing and retreating you can find the opponent's defects and establish your own superior position." If one part moves and the other parts do not move, the whole body will be in confusion.

7. Insubstantial and substantial must be clearly differentiated.

When practicing T'ai Chi it is of the utmost importance to discriminate between the insubstantial and substantial aspects. For instance, if the whole body's weight is on the right foot, the right foot is substantial and the left foot is insubstantial, and vice versa. If one can discriminate between the insubstantial and substantial, the movement of steps and turning of the body will be light and nimble. Otherwise they will be heavy and clumsy, and you will be uprooted with a slight pull and push by your opponent. If you want to step forward with your right foot, you must shift your entire weight to the left foot and leave no weight on the right foot —then the movement will be light and agile. When you (try to) step forward with one foot while there is still some weight on both feet, it is called double-weighting. The movement will be heavy and clumsy and put you into a posture "ready to be beaten." It is said in the T'ai Chi Classics: "The insubstantial and substantial must be clearly discriminated. Every part of the body has both a substantial and insubstantial aspect at any given time. The entire body also has this feature if considered as one unit."

8. Concentrate the line of vision.

Your eyes must look forward to an imaginary opponent in front of you, watching him constantly to see what he will do to you. When your body turns in one direction, your eyes must look forward in the same direction. It is incorrect to look toward the Southeast by turning your head while your body is facing East. The head and body should be considered as one unit.

9. All the movements must be connected without severance. When the energy is severed, use mind-intent to reconnect it.

All the postures are to be practiced slowly, effortlessly, and continuously so that the ch'i and blood can circulate through the entire body without hindrance. Suppose one posture contains four beats—you must stop momentarily at the end of the fourth beat to complete the movement of the posture, then go on to another posture. So during the transition from one posture to another, you must stop for just half a second. This momentary stoppage will be connected and joined to the next posture by the mind-intent. If one goes on to another posture before the preceding one is fully completed, this is not the correct way of "continuously moving." It is confusion, and one will not be able to determine clearly which of the postures is which. The Classics say: "T'ai Chi Ch'uan is also called 'Chang Ch'uan' (Long Boxing) because it flows unceasingly like the great river." The great T'ai Chi Master Lao Chen said, "The energy breaks off, but is joined and connected by the mind-intent, just as the lotus root is broken but the fibers remain connected."

10. Meditation in action.

In other kinds of boxing arts, one must use tremendous external muscular force. This results in the expansion of veins and blood vessels, impediment of the ch'i, exhaustion, and panting, all of which are bad for health. When practicing T'ai Chi you must control your movements by tranquillity and direct the movements by mind-intent rather than by external muscular force. Then the movements will be effortless, continuous, and slow. The slower one practices (without stopping or jerking) the better. Gradually the above mentioned defects will be eliminated. If the student ponders the matter carefully, he will be able to grasp the idea and acquire the beauty of this art without difficulty.

8
Discussion of the Mind-Intent and the Ch'i

The mind and ch'i in man's body are formless, colorless, and invisible. We must realize that the ch'i occupies a most important place in the body because it gives the blood impetus to circulate freely and nourishes the blood in order to replenish and strengthen the body. The ch'i is developed by cherishing and nurturing the fire of the kidneys *(ming men huo)* and the reproductive secretions. The Taoists called this "water and fire in coordination" or the "internal elixer (of immortality)." It is preserved in the tan t'ien, a point 1 1/3 inches below the navel. The Taoists treasured it most dearly. Ordinarily people think that the blood is the most precious substance in the body, but in reality the ch'i is of greater value than the blood because the ch'i is the master and the blood is the assistant. The ch'i protects the blood and the blood nourishes the body. Man's whole life depends on this protection and nourishment. If there is only nourishment without protection there will be no circulation of the blood; if there is only protection without nourishment there will be no harmony. In other words, protection is of the utmost importance and nourishment is secondary. A person can live for a time with insufficient blood, but with insufficient ch'i one is in imminent danger of death. So the cultivation of the ch'i is of prime importance.

The special feature of T'ai Chi Ch'uan is that in addition to nurturing the body, it emphasizes especially cultivation of the ch'i. As the saying goes, "Externally strengthen your muscles, bones, and skin. Internally develop and fill up your ch'i." Anyone who practices T'ai Chi Ch'uan will find that after doing the postures Pushing Hands or Ta Lü, the breathing is still natural, the countenance has not changed, and the ch'i within is circulating freely through the entire body, so that one feels much more comfortable than before practicing. It is evident that if one can cultivate the ch'i the beneficial effects will be great indeed and the defects of haste and weariness will not occur. Furthermore, when the ch'i is properly nurtured the (constituents of the) blood will be sufficient; when the blood is sufficient the body will be strong; when the body is strong the mind will be firm and sincere; when the mind is firm and sincere the sentient soul *(po)* will be vigorous so that one can prolong life and find the way to immortality.

Although some say that the heart (mind) and the intention are identical, there is a difference. The mind is the master and the intention is the assistant. When the mind moves, the mind-intent is immediately aroused; when the intent is aroused, the ch'i will immediately follow. So the heart (mind), the intent, and the ch'i are closely connected like a circle. When the mind is confused, the intention will be dispersed and when the intention is dispersed the ch'i will float upward. On the contrary, when the ch'i sinks to the tan t'ien the mind-intent will be firm and sincere; when the mind-intent is firm and sincere, the mind (heart) will be tranquil. So the three are interdependent, closely related, and inseparable from one another. When the ch'i can circulate throughout the entire body without hindrance it will expedite the movement of the blood and also mobilize the spirit of vitality. When one reaches this stage, then one can apply the art in functional use. For the mind-intent and the ch'i are the principles and the techniques (or the postures) are the methods. If one has only principles without techniques, one will never acquire a wide and far-reaching insight; to have only techniques without principles is like forsaking the roots and clinging to the topmost branches. Therefore there is a close connection and mutual relationship between the mind-intent and the ch'i and the techniques found in the postures.

Although making use of the mind-intent and the ch'i is quite difficult for beginners in T'ai Chi Ch'uan, it is by no means impossible to do so. When one begins to practice the thirteen postures or practices postures singly, one must start out by having the concept of "imagination" always in mind. For example, when both hands form the posture of "Push," you must pretend that there is an opponent in front of you. At this time you may not (yet) be able to issue ch'i from your palms. But you continue to imagine the ch'i emanating from the tan t'ien, adhering to the spine, then being mobilized through the back to the arms, wrists, and palms, and finally issuing outward from the palms to the imaginary opponent's body. When beginners practice, this type of "imagination" is indistinct and vague, but if they practice over a long period of time, they will be able to use this at will and the "imagination" will become a reality.

When the ch'i circulates throughout the entire body without hindrance, the feelings and perceptions of the body, the muscles, and the touch become sensitive and alert. The spirit of vitality becomes lively and clear. When one employs external muscular exertion to practice T'ai Chi, the ch'i will be impeded or will float upwards. When one becomes angry, the ch'i will become coarse and harsh. These types of ch'i cannot produce a powerful intrinsic energy, nor can they cause the feet to become firmly rooted. Moreover, they are detrimental to health. The ch'i which is produced from correct T'ai Chi practice is entirely different. It emanates from the tan t'ien and is peaceful and clear. When the ch'i is peaceful and clear, it will be harmonious; when it is in harmony, it will circulate through the whole body without impediment. When one practices T'ai Chi the entire body must be completely relaxed, the mind should be concentrated, and the movement should be slow, effortless, continuously flowing, light and nimble. Only by practicing T'ai Chi in this manner can you let your ch'i sink deeply to the tan t'ien.

In the T'ai Chi Classic known as "The Mental Elucidation of the Thirteen Postures," there are many passages relating to the ch'i:

"Let the mind direct the ch'i so that it sinks deeply and steadily and can permeate the bones. Let the ch'i circulate throughout the entire body freely and without hindrance so that the body will follow the dictates of the mind."

"The mind and the ch'i must respond ingeniously and efficaciously to the exchange of substantial and insubstantial so as to develop an active and harmonious tendency."

"To direct the ch'i is like threading a pearl with nine crooked paths. There is no hollow which it does not penetrate."

"The ch'i should be cultivated naturally and harmoniously so as to avoid ill effects."

"The mind is the commander; the ch'i is the banner."

"The abdomen is completely relaxed, enabling the ch'i to penetrate the bones."

"When you push and pull, withdraw and attack, your ch'i adheres to the back of your body."

In the "Song of the Substance and Function of the Thirteen Postures," it says:

"Ch'i will circulate throughout the entire body without the slightest hindrance."

"When the abdomen is completely relaxed, the ch'i will soar up (and circulate throughout the entire body)."

"The mind and ch'i direct and the flesh and bones follow."

All of the above passages emphasize the importance of the ch'i. It is entirely up to the student to discriminate whether the ch'i is peaceful and clear or clumsy and violent. The peaceful and clear ch'i should be acquired and the clumsy and violent ch'i must be avoided.

9
Slowness and Non-exertion of Muscular Force

The movement of T'ai Chi Ch'uan should be slow, and external muscular force should not be used. Many students harbor doubts about this principle—they think that T'ai Chi can be good for health but cannot be put to practical use. The method of practice in T'ai Chi is to study the principles first; when the principles have been thoroughly understood one learns specific techniques; when the techniques have been thoroughly mastered, then they can be applied in practical use. It is not because the art cannot be employed in practical use that students harbor doubts, but because their mastery of techniques has not yet reached the proper level. The process is like the refining of steel: starting with iron ore, one melts it into cast iron; from cast iron into wrought iron; and from wrought iron into pure steel. If it has not passed through a long period of refining time, it will be of no use.

The reason that one can acquire the art of T'ai Chi by slow motion is that its practice is based entirely upon the natural way, not stressing external muscular force and holding of the breath, but emphasizing the use of the mind to direct all movements. Using external muscular force makes movement clumsy; holding the breath hinders the circulation of the blood. Therefore it is of the utmost importance to sink the ch'i to the tan t'ien and completely relax the entire body, without exerting the slightest energy. The principle of T'ai Chi is to control action by tranquillity and to conquer the forceful and unyielding with the gentle and yielding. From nothingness something is produced: it looks like nothing, though it is something; it looks soft, but in reality it is firm.

When an adverse situation comes about, one must adapt to it by yielding without hitch or hindrance, without letting go and with no resistance. These are all variations of substantial and insubstantial. Slow means leisurely and gradual. Because the movement is slow, it is tranquil; because it is tranquil, the ch'i can sink deeply to the tan t'ien and abide there; when the ch'i can sink deeply and abide in the tan t'ien, then one can maintain oneself firmly. This is called the central equilibrium of mind and ch'i. When the mind can be maintained firmly, then a calm unperturbedness can be attained; and to that calmness there will succeed a tranquil repose of the spirit of vitality. After one has achieved a tranquil repose of the spirit of vitality, then the ch'i can sink to the tan t'ien. When the ch'i has sunk deeply to the tan t'ien, then the spirit of vitality will be concentrated so that one can have concentration of attention and energy, and circulation of ch'i throughout the entire body without hindrance.

Slowness comes from the mind's being delicate and careful; when the mind is delicate and careful, then the spirit will be clear; when the spirit of vitality is clear, the ch'i will be vigorous, and the defect of a hindrance to the circulation of ch'i will be no more.

Fast motion comes from carelessness and giddiness of the mind. Carelessness and giddiness of the mind come from haste. When the mind is in haste, the ch'i will be floating upward; when the ch'i is floating upward it will not sink deeply in the tan t'ien. When the mind is in haste, it cannot be quiet and tranquil. When the ch'i cannot sink and the mind is not tranquil, the mind will have nothing by which to abide. Then the whole body will be in disorder and confusion, and it will be impossible to obtain lightness and agility.

To control action by tranquillity and conquer the hard with the soft arc functions of the feelings and sensibility of the body and mind. Therefore the practice of the postures of T'ai Chi is intended to discipline the body and mind for health. The techniques which are applied in functional use are from Pushing Hands. The first step of Pushing Hands is to make a thorough investigation of feeling and sensibility. When the body is affected by a movement, the mind is immediately aware of it. The sensibility is so refined and subtle that the functional use is unlimited and inexhaustible. Therefore one is able to know his own plans and to be acquainted with those of his opponent: their taste and flavor can be obtained from the apprehension and comprehension of the mind and spirit of vitality. It is impossible to describe this in words. The inexhaustibility of the changes and variations is the result of the alertness of feelings and sensibility. Thus one can detect substantial and insubstantial and reach a state of total reliance on the mind. This is the real significance of the slow movement and non-exertion of muscular force.

When practicing the postures of T'ai Chi, one should perform the movements as slowly as possible. When they are put to practical use, they are not slow at all. In the Classics it is said: "To withdraw means to attack, and to yield is also to strike." The actions of withdrawal and attack arise at the same time, and the movements of yield and strike happen simultaneously. It is like a lever system in physics.

It is my opinion that when one has mastered the techniques of Roll Back ([Lü] and Receiving Energy [chieh chin]), one has already acquired the art of T'ai Chi and reached the highest level. Usually the Roll Back technique is called "to open the door and welcome the robber in." Of course, if you don't open the door the robber cannot take anything from you, and you also cannot catch him. When your opponent strikes you with his fist you have to use the Roll Back technique to yield and neutralize his striking force so that he cannot catch you. For this you must have the technique of equilibrium so that you can direct your waist to yield and neutralize the striking force, otherwise your waist will not obey your order. Next you have to strike immediately and catch the opponent ("yield means attack" technique). This is not an easy matter. You must discover his defects and your own superior position, avoid being double-weighted, and concentrate single-mindedly on his center of gravity, his straight line, his substantial and insubstantial, employing your whole body as one unit. When you have all these techniques in your mind before giving expression to them, your attack will be effective and you will surely catch your opponent.

Once you have acquired this Roll Back technique, we can talk about the second technique, which is Receiving Energy. This energy is like the penalty kick in a soccer game. The shooting of the ball is so fast and hard that the goalkeeper has to stretch out his hands and body to meet it and immediately withdraw in order to neutralize the fast and hard force so that he can catch the ball easily in his hands. If he collides with the ball (force against force), the ball will fly away and the goalkeeper will be hurt besides. The receiving energy technique of T'ai Chi is even more difficult than the goalkeeper's handling of the ball. When your opponent attacks you with a hundred pounds of energy, wait until he has spent half of it and has only fifty pounds left, and then counterattack immediately. It will be as though he has been hit by a thunderbolt, and he will be pushed far, far away. How crucial it is to calculate accurately the timing, velocity, strength, and direction of the opponent!

10
Secrets
(the Secret Technique)
of the Eight Postures

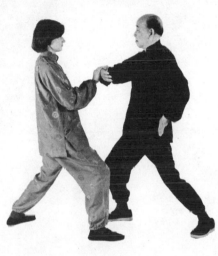

1.

What is the meaning of "Ward Off" energy?
It is like the water supporting a moving boat.
First one must sink ch'i to the tan t'ien (fill
　　the tan t'ien up with ch'i),
then one must hold the head as if suspended from
　　above.
The entire body is full of springlike energy,
　　opening and closing in a very quick moment.
Even if there is an opposing force of one
　　thousand pounds,
One can uproot the opponent and make him float
　　without difficulty.

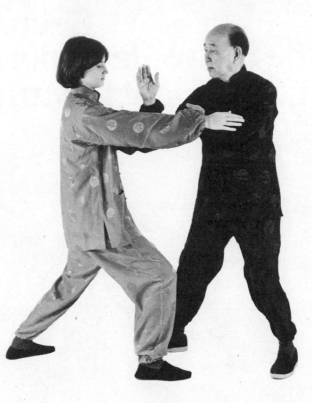

2.

What is the meaning of "Roll Back" energy?
Entice the opponent, make him come forward,
    go along with his incoming energy
    lightly and nimbly without letting go and with
    no resistance.
When his force is used to the extreme degree, it
    will naturally become empty.
One can now let (the opponent) go or counter at
    will.
Maintain your own equilibrium and you will not be
    able to be taken advantage of by others.

78

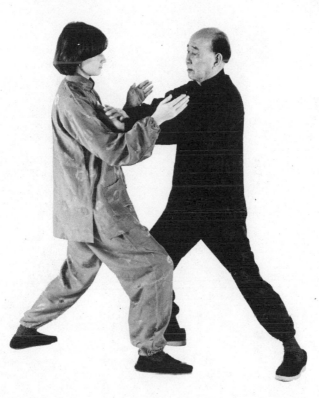

3.

What is the meaning of "Press" energy?
In functional use there are two aspects:

(a) The direct way is a simple concept . . .
Going to meet the opponent and closing
(attaching gently) are one action.
(b) The indirect way is the reaction force . . .
like the rebound of a ball hitting a wall or of a
coin thrown on a drumhead, bouncing off with
a ringing sound.

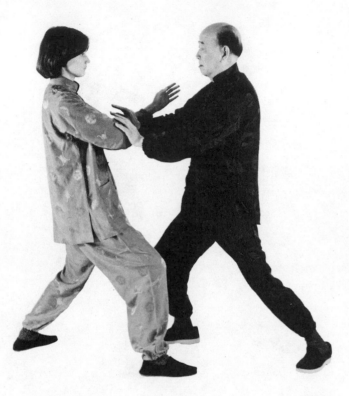

4.

What is the meaning of "Push" energy?
When mobilizing energy it is like flowing water.
The substantial is concealed in the insubstantial.
The power of the turbulent flow is difficult to
    resist.
Coming to a high place, it swells and fills the place
    up;
meeting a hollow it dives downward.
There are troughs and crests in the waves.
There is no opening into which it does not enter.

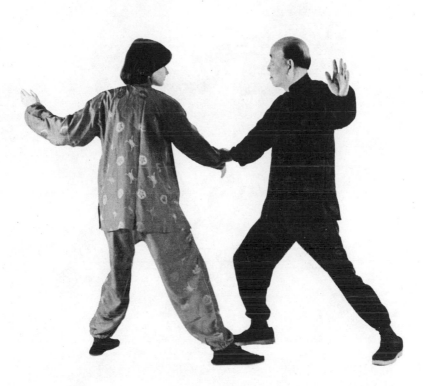

5.

What is the meaning of "Pull" energy?

It is like a weight attached to the beam of a
    steelyard.

No matter how heavy or light the force is,
    you will find out how heavy or light it is
    after weighing it.

To push and pull requires only four ounces . . .

One thousand pounds can also be balanced.

If you ask what the principle is,
    the answer is the function of the lever.

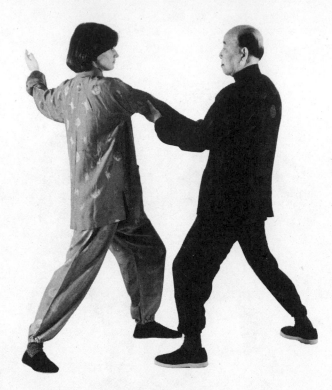

6.

What is the meaning of "Split" energy?
It revolves like a spinning disc.
If something is thrown onto it,
    it will immediately be cast more than ten feet
    away.
Did you not see the whirlpool?
The waves roll in spiraling currents . . .
The falling leaves drop into it
    and suddenly sink and disappear.

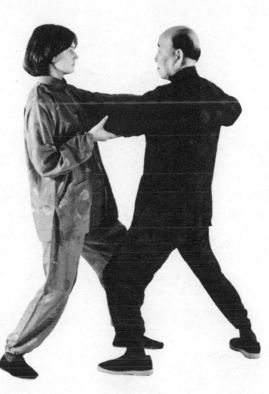

7.

What is the meaning of "Elbow-Stroke" energy?
The method relates to the Five Elements.
Yin and Yang are differentiated as to
 high and low.
Substantial and Insubstantial must be clearly
 discriminated.
Joined in unbroken continuity, the posture cannot ·
 be resisted.
The chopping fist is especially fearsome.
After one has thoroughly understood the six kinds
 of energy,
 the functional use becomes unlimited.

Note: In this stanza, the energy of "Elbow-Stroke" includes the technique
of the chopping fist. The elbow and the fist can work in alternation.

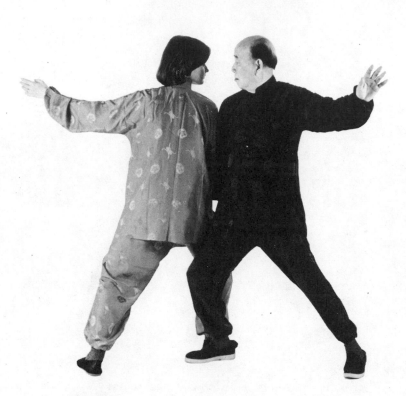

8.

What is the meaning of "Shoulder-Stroke" energy?
Its method is divided into shoulder and back
    technique.
In diagonal flying posture use shoulder,
    but within the shoulder technique, there is also
    some use of back.
Once you have the chance and the posture,
    the technique explodes like pounding a pestle.
Carefully maintain your own center of gravity.
If you lose it, the technique is of no avail.

11
Detailed Explanation of the Essential Meaning of the Five Elements

The Five Elements are: Metal, Wood, Water, Fire, and Earth. The energies of the Five Elements are: *Adhere, Join, Stick to, Follow, and Do not let go and do not resist.* We will now explain each kind of energy in detail:

1. *Adhere* is exemplified in two things coming into contact, one with the other: they adhere, and the lower one is lifted up. In T'ai Chi technical terms this is called intrinsic energy. This kind of energy does not pull up directly, but is developed indirectly. It consists of the principles of energy and mental intent both working together. If in Pushing Hands or combat an opponent's physique is very powerful and his strength is abundant, his stance very firm and stable so that it is difficult to make him lose balance or shift his center of gravity, then by using "adhere" energy one can cause him to lose his own center of gravity. Use mind-intent to test him; make his ch'i rise upward, his entire spirit of vitality concentrate upward so that his body is heavy but his legs light; then his root will naturally be broken—this is caused by his reaction force. Then withdraw the hands slightly in accordance with his movement and, using

the energy of "not letting go and not resisting," induce him to be suspended and empty. This is called "adhere" energy.

This energy is like adhering to and lifting up a ball. During the moment of laying hands on it and lifting it, if one can apply this technique perfectly, the ball will not leave the hand. Adhere and then lift. This is what is expressed in the saying, "To adhere is to retreat; to retreat is called adhering."

The mental conception is a kind of imagination. Using the principle of substantial and insubstantial, one sees to it that the opponent is completely unsuspecting, and strikes him when he is altogether unprepared. Even if the opponent has plenty of real power and defends himself vigilantly, not afraid of being attacked and not afraid of an opponent's strong force, nevertheless he is very much afraid that an opponent may try to trick him. If I lure him with a bait and make him abandon his defensive position to take up an offensive one, then his real power will disperse. I take this opportunity to find out his defect and strike him. This is to entice and uproot him.

Thus he falls into a snare through his own fault. This is called attacking when he is not in a defensive position, but keeping one's own defensive position even when the opponent is apparently not in an offensive position. The T'ai Chi Classics say: "If your opponent does not move, you should not move. At his slightest stir you have already anticipated it and are able to move first." This expresses the same principle as the entire discussion above.

The student must constantly investigate this and comprehend it. After a long time it will manifest itself naturally.

2. *Join* means to go through and connect together: not to break off in the middle, not to slip off—to attach continuously without pause, without stopping, without rest. This is called "join" energy.

3. *Stick to* means to fasten on and stick. If the opponent advances, I retreat; if he retreats, I advance. If he "floats," I follow up immediately. If he sinks, I relax. If he tries to let go,

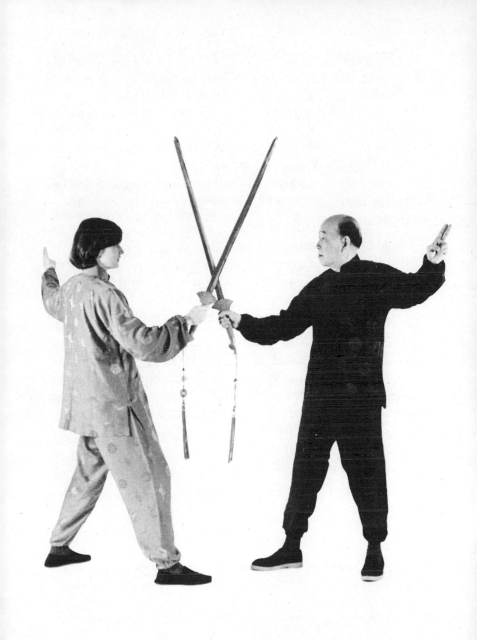

I immediately fill in the gap and he cannot get rid of me. If he tries to push forward ("throw me away"), his energy cannot come to my body so I do not go away. It is like pasting on and sticking, without letting go and with no resistance. This is called "sticking" energy.

The T'ai Chi Classics say: "When he pushes upward or downward against you he feels as if there is no end to the emptiness he encounters. When he advances against you he feels the distance incredibly long; when he retreats he feels it exasperatingly short."

4. *Follow* means to obey. Whether the opponent is slow or quick, you must respond accordingly. When he advances or retreats, you must comply. One must not let go or separate, not move first nor move last, neither too soon nor too late. Give up your own initiative and follow that of others. This is called "following" energy.

5. *Do not let go and do not resist.* To let go means to open a gap. To resist means to collide. Do not come apart; do not struggle against; do not strive to be first; do not fall behind. The source of the Five Elements, the foundation of lightness and agility, this is called "not letting go and not resisting."

12
(T'ai Chi Ch'uan) Song of Pushing Hands, with Explanatory Comments

In Ward Off, Roll Back, Press, and Push one must know the correct technique.

Ward Off, Roll Back, Press, and Push are the four cardinal points (directions). They are supplemented by the movements of the four corners—Pull, Split, Elbow-Stroke, and Shoulder-Stroke. Together, all of these are called the Eight Positions (openings), and all the variations in T'ai Chi Ch'uan are derived from them. The four methods of Ward Off, Roll Back, Press, and Push are the basis of all the techniques. They cannot be diminished, nor can they be altered. One must differentiate clearly between them, and know where to find their true meaning. If one cannot discern these fundamental methods clearly, then how can one be qualified to speak of T'ai Chi Ch'uan? If one should put forth strenuous mental effort for a long time, it would still be to no avail; for even after one has understood the true meaning of the four cardinal points, if one knows only how to make empty talk about theory it will still be of no practical use whatever. So one must sit and discuss them, then get up and put them into practice. Only by constant study and practice can one have any hope of success.

The lower and upper parts of the body must act in unison, so that an opponent would find it difficult to advance and attack.

From the foot to the leg to the waist, from the shoulder to the hand to the fingers, from the lower part to the upper part— all must act as one unit. No matter whether it is in the hand, the body, or the foot, the movement must be active and alert so that it can be applied at will. All the parts of the body, from head to toe, must correspond with each other so that an opponent has no opportunity to take advantage and would find it difficult to advance and attack.

Even though he should come to attack with great force . . .

Even if one is attacked with great force, there is no need to be afraid. One must control his mind, like a commanding general —if Mt. T'ai were to collapse in front of him, his expression would not change.

Use a push and pull of four ounces to deflect a momentum of one thousand pounds.

When the opponent comes to attack with the force of one thousand pounds, his energy can be deflected with a force of four ounces. The reason this can be done is not the energy of the four ounces, but the power of push-pull. When the opponent strikes with a force of one thousand pounds, he comes in a straight line; if one meets him with the body facing directly forward, then the difference between the superior and defective positions is very great. If one attempts to deflect one thousand pounds with a force of one thousand pounds, there is still doubt as to who will win; and even if one *can* deflect it, it still means that one thousand pounds must be used to deflect one thousand pounds. One must move in accordance with the opponent's incoming posture and apply the technique of pull and push: *then* one can use four ounces to deflect a momentum of one thousand pounds. However, the size of the deflecting force, and the direction of the deflecting movement, must be decided by a clear observation of the energy, velocity, and direction of the opponent's incoming posture. One cannot deal with all situations in the same manner or settle the matter with one simple deflection movement. If one uses excessive or insufficient energy, or if the direction is too straight or too much inclined to the side, one will fall into the errors of letting go or resisting, and then no technique can be applied successfully. The student should not take this as something to talk about easily or to look at lightly. In fact, it appears easy, but to practice it is quite difficult. Only after learning how to interpret energy *(tung chin)* can one be qualified to speak about it.

Entice him to advance; when his energy is emptied, adhere to him and issue energy.

If the opponent maintains a firm attitude, not committing himself, it is very difficult to find an opportunity to attack. In such a situation one can deliberately expose one's weak point, and being ready beforehand, entice him to advance and attack. The opponent's attack will have to become empty. (As one deftly evades an opponent's attack, his attacking limb will naturally meet nothing but emptiness, and he will be temporarily thrown off balance.) Taking advantage of the moment when he has not yet recovered his steady stance, one uses the body as a unit, mobilizes the energy, and strikes. As soon as energy is issued, the opponent is propelled away. An expert strategist often uses an empty camp to lure the enemy, waits until the enemy attacks the empty place, and then attacks him with concealed troops. This is the meaning of all of the above.

Further Commentary:

Ho chi ch'u (合即出) means that one adheres to him and issues energy. "Ho" indicates adhering gently to the opponent, feeling his strong and weak points. Also, before issuing energy, one must know the opponent's center of gravity and the most effective line in which to attack him. One must not be double-weighted, but must relax and concentrate all energy in one direction. If these conditions are not met, then one will make a "blind push," which cannot be effective. Before issuing energy one must have all these principles clearly in mind.

Adhere, join, stick to, and follow with no letting go and with no resistance.

"Adhere" means to lift and pull up, so that the opponent's heel leaves the ground (he is uprooted) and his stance "floats" unsteadily. "Join" means to give up oneself and not leave the other—that is, to "forget the self and follow the other." "Stick to" means to struggle to remain attached, not allowing the opponent to separate himself and escape. "Follow" means that when the opponent moves away, one must adapt to his movement, following his movements in any situation. The four techniques above all involve "not letting go and not resisting." No letting go, in this case, is not allowing the opponent to detach himself and escape, but keeping him constantly under control. Not resisting, in this case, is not giving the opponent an opportunity to issue his hidden energy. He has no way to apply his techniques (art). Adhere, join, stick, and follow, without letting go and with no resistance, are exceedingly fine and delicate techniques. One must study and examine them very thoroughly. Only if one seeks diligently to assimilate the information contained herein will he be able to understand.

When one has been struck and is just about to fall over, he must hop like a sparrow.

A common saying has it: "A man may lose control of his hand, while a horse may stumble." At the moment when one is facing an opponent one may find oneself in an inferior position which one cannot avoid. If one should be in such a situation, one's mind must not become confused and flustered. When one is just about to be struck and there is no time to avoid it, one must imitate the hopping of a sparrow. Both feet leave the ground simultaneously and jump away at once, to prevent a fall. After this jumping, the body is not scattered but still acts as a unit, and the mind and spirit are not confused. If the opponent continues to advance and attack, the situation can be dealt with in a calm and unruffled manner.

If the opponent uses the press technique very efficiently, one's body must act in the most suitable manner when escaping.

During the critical moment of being pressed by the opponent, if one wishes to escape he must use the body, as a unit, in the most appropriate manner: it should be "empty" and receptive, with energy concealed within—not hard or tense—to neutralize the opponent's pressing energy. At the same time, both hands must be placed forward to control the opponent and to meet his next attack.

Hold the back erect, let the chest be relaxed and "hollow," as in the Concluding Form of T'ai Chi.

"Hold the back erect and hollow the chest" resembles the posture in the Concluding Form of T'ai Chi. This is a posture in which one reserves one's own energy internally, while waiting for the opponent to issue his. This is what the Classics call "the appearance of a hawk about to seize a rabbit and the spirit of a cat catching a rat."

Cover the groin, protect the "kidneys," and take steps in accordance with the Five Elements.

"Cover the groin" means that the toes of the front foot must turn slightly inward, with both knees slightly bent inward in order to protect the "kidneys."* The Five Elements and the steps in accordance with the Five Elements are Advance, Retreat, Look to the Left, Gaze Right, and Central Equilibrium. These are the fundamental steps of the art of T'ai Chi Ch'uan. In Central Equilibrium one stands firmly rooted so

* The Chinese character for "kidneys" can also refer to the male organs.

that one can take steps to the left or right and advance or retreat at will.

When the student has thoroughly comprehended the meaning of all the above statements, he will be able to understand quickly and completely the marvelous technique of the entire body.

Concerning what is said above, one must pay particular attention to the two statements: "In Ward Off, Roll Back, Press, and Push, one must know the correct technique" and "Adhere, join, stick to, and follow, with no letting go and with no resistance." But without a long period of practice and study it is not easy to comprehend these techniques thoroughly.

When the T'ai Chi techniques have been mastered, their marvels are amazing. The fame of the former Master Yang Lu Chan in Peking spread near and far, and he was often visited by experts in the martial arts. One day when he was quietly sitting, a monk arrived unexpectedly. The Master went out to welcome him and noted his strong and imposing physique—he stood some seven feet tall. When he had bowed and paid his compliments, the Master replied very courteously and modestly. Later, while they were conversing in the Master's house, the monk suddenly jumped up and punched the Master with the speed of a hawk pouncing on its prey. The Master hollowed his chest slightly, using his right palm to stop the oncoming fist; then he lightly patted it. The monk, as if receiving an electric shock, fell behind the decorative screen, his fist still extended. Then, regaining his composure, he begged the Master to forgive his rudeness. The Master invited him to chat.

The monk accepted and repeatedly inquired as to why his unexpected attack had not fulfilled its purpose. The Master replied that this was called "taking heed at every moment." Then the monk inquired about why he had fallen with such speed. The Master replied, "This is known as 'Issuing energy like shooting an arrow.'" The monk said, "I have traveled the entire realm and I have never met another like you, Master." He then insistently asked about the miracle of T'ai Chi's "lightness and agility." The Master was just about to answer when a swallow entered through the curtain, flying low and circling near his body. He suddenly shot out his hand and caught it. Looking at the monk, he said, "This bird is very tame and follows a man's will, so I shall play with it." He supported it on his right palm and stroked it with his left hand. Then he withdrew his left hand. The swallow spread its wings, ready to fly. The Master's palm stirred ever so slightly, its energy "suddenly concealed, suddenly manifest." The swallow was unable to fly away after all. For any bird, no matter what its kind, must use the stretching energy of its feet in order to help its body take off. The swallow's feet had no place to exert strength; therefore, even though it had wings, it could not fly away. The swallow seemed already tamed, so the Master again stroked it to make it go; but again it could not take off. This happened three times. The monk exclaimed, "This art—how marvelous it is!" The Master laughed and replied, "This is not worthy of being called marvelous. When one has practiced T'ai Chi for a long time and the entire body has become light and agile, then the weight of a feather cannot be added nor can a fly alight." The monk acknowledged the Master's superiority. He remained and talked for three days before he left.

The above is a record of fact, and the student should not regard it as a false story purporting to be history. One's intention must be to learn from the highest. Only then will one's skill arrive naturally at an advanced stage.

If the opponent does not move, I do not move . . .

"If the opponent does not move, I do not move" means that one remains at ease yet alert until the opponent puts forth his energy. The explanation of T'ai Chi principles says, "Remain tranquil while waiting for movement. When the opportunity comes, then attack immediately." This is the proper way to act. To put out one's hands in a hasty and confused manner, looking high and low for an opportunity to strike the opponent, is far from the correct method. This principle is quite obvious.

Some say, if the opponent does not move at all, then what should one do? In this case one can stretch out a hand in a false attack to draw on the opponent once, twice, or three times; then he cannot but move. If he persists in not moving, the feint can immediately be changed into a real attack, taking advantage of the situation and leaving the opponent at a loss as to how to respond, with no way to avoid the attack.

If the opponent moves even slightly, I move first.

When one "joins hands" with an opponent, one does not make the first move. One's spirit must pay close attention and remain alert, waiting for the moment when the opponent is just about to move. Then, one's hand has already moved before he does. But the difference in time between "slightly moving" and "already having moved" is the time of the blink of an eye. If there is the slightest delay, the chance will be lost. If the hand is stretched out a little too slowly and the opponent has already moved, then even if one should want to move first, it is quite impossible. This must be clearly perceived.

The energy appears "relaxed," but is not so relaxed.

When one is practicing in accordance with the principles of T'ai Chi, one's movement appears relaxed, but in reality is not so relaxed. This expression is basically obvious and simple, but it can very easily be misinterpreted, for the movements of most beginners are tense and stiff and the teacher uses the word "relax" to correct this. While the student is tense, he must pay attention to relaxing. But the relaxation needed is a relative quality, not an absolute one. It is like the undulating motion of a snake—sometimes it raises its head, sometimes it coils itself up. At every moment one can see its energy concealed internally. This is what is meant by appearing "relaxed," but not so relaxed. If one relaxes to the stage of collapse, then the intrinsic energy will be entirely absent, as in a dead snake lying on the ground. But the extent to which one appears "relaxed" but is not so relaxed, must be conceived mentally; it cannot be expressed in words. If the student will diligently remember this rule, in time he will come to understand it for himself.

About to extend, but not yet fully extended . . .

The foot and hand movements of T'ai Chi, extending or stretching out, always take as their standard: "almost straight, but not completely straightened." If the movements are straightened to the extreme, then one's energy will be exhausted. When this principle is applied to the hand, most beginners will understand how to do it; but when it is applied to the legs, they will frequently misinterpret (and fail to heed) the correct principle. The movement of the steps in T'ai Chi does not go beyond bending the leg and sitting back on it; each movement mutually interchanges with the other. If the forward leg is bent, the rear leg is straightened; if the rear leg is sitting back, the front leg is straightened. The word "straightened" is a relative term, not an absolute one. When teaching, the former masters would often say only the one word "straight" in order to simplify. What they said is not incorrect, but if one took this as the rule, one might well make a wrong interpretation.

Now we will provide an example to make the matter clear. Among the postures which sit back on the leg, such as Lift Hands, Play Lute, Squatting Single Whip, etc., the forward leg must be slightly bent and not entirely straightened or stretched out; otherwise not only will the forward leg be clumsy and lack agility, but if one is pulled or pushed even slightly, the entire body will be shaken. The influence of this will reach the point where the ch'i in the entire body will be obstructed and will not flow smoothly. If the student examines this thoroughly, he will see that what we say is not incorrect.

As far as the bent leg is concerned, in the forward "Bow Stance," whether one practices the postures, Pushing Hands, or engages in combat, the rear leg must not be completely straightened out. If the rear leg is stretched out to the extreme point, there will be no energy left to issue.

The T'ai Chi Classics say, "Seek the straight in the curved." The Classics again say, "If one cannot obtain a favorable opportunity or a superior position, one's body will be disordered and in confusion. To correct this fault, one must adjust the waist and legs." The student must give this saying his repeated consideration.

The energy may be broken off, but the [mind]-intention is not broken off.

After issuing energy, one's hand is stretched out. The energy is already broken off, but the mind-intention is not yet broken off, so that one can change in accordance with the circumstances continuously and without impediment. An old master said, "The energy may be broken off, but the mind intent is not broken off. The lotus root may be broken, but the inner tissues are not broken off." This is the meaning of the above.

First in the mind, then in the body . . .

The beginner must use and concentrate his mind when facing an opponent, but he may not be able to overcome the opponent . . . When one has fully mastered the art, one need not use the mind. When one is attacked, one can automatically adapt to the situation and respond to the attack. One's mind is not even aware of it, but the attacker has already been propelled away without one's being aware of how one's hand was used. Beginners must rely on the mind; when one has fully mastered the art, one can rely on the body. It is like a beginner learning the abacus. At first he must recite the formulas while counting and using his hand. Later, when he has mastered the abacus, his hand can act at will, even though his mind is no longer preoccupied with the formulas. This is what is meant by "First in the mind, then in the body."

Note —Concerning "First in the mind, then in the body," there is the famous story of Yang Ch'eng Fu. Strolling with his disciples one day on the outskirts of a city, Yang was unexpectedly struck from the rear by a rickshaw. The rickshaw with its occupants rebounded off Yang's body and was propelled ten feet away. The Master, hardly aware of the incident, continued his conversation as if nothing untoward had happened.—*Ed.*

The abdomen is completely relaxed—then the ch'i can permeate the bones; the spirit is at ease and the body is tranquil.

Although one concentrates on the abdomen, it must nevertheless be relaxed and at ease. One must not hold or force one's energy. When the ch'i sinks and permeates the bones, they become heavy. Externally one feels soft as cotton; internally one feels like an iron bar. One is like an iron bar wrapped in cotton. Externally one is soft and supple; internally one is firm.

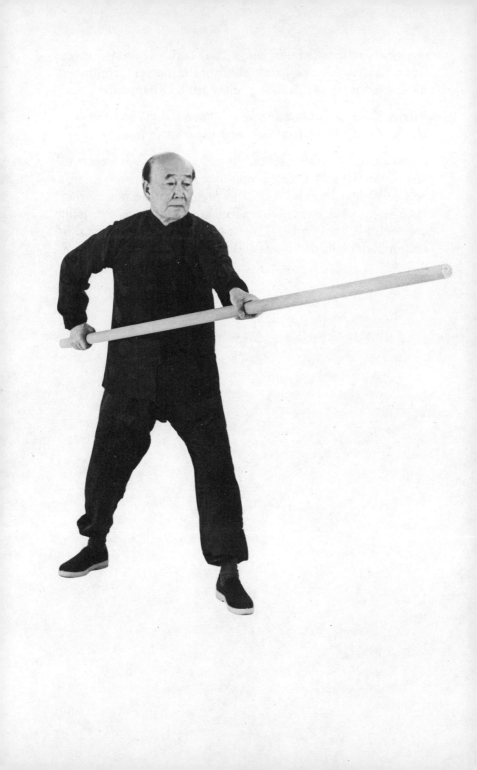

13
Other
Short Texts

Some of these texts have not been given here in their entirety because much of the material duplicates that in other sections of this book. Therefore, only those parts of these texts that convey some new insight have been rendered here.—*Ed.*

Central Equilibrium

The condition before one has stretched out, contracted, opened, or closed is called centrality. Remaining still without motion is called equilibrium. The mind is clear and the ch'i harmonious; the spirit of vitality rises to the top of the head while one neither leans nor inclines—this is called the ch'i of central equilibrium. This is also the basic principle of the way to immortality.

The Light and Alert Energy on the Top of the Head

The energy of holding up the head is like being suspended from above. When the top of the head is erect and the abdomen is completely relaxed, the ch'i sinks to the tan t'ien and the spirit of vitality reaches to the top of the head. It is like a weighted doll—the top part is light and the bottom part heavy, or like a buoy floating on the water, drifting hither and thither without thinking.

The song says, "The clear spirit of vitality and deeply sinking ch'i maintain their natural aspect. Drifting hither and thither, diving into the waves, let the wind and waves hit you and blow you; your top is light, your bottom heavy; you cannot be overturned."

Feeling and Sensibility

What the body feels, the mind senses. Where there is feeling, there is response. Every movement creates feeling; when there is feeling there is response; after response, there is again a feeling of responding; after this feeling of responding, there is another response. Thus, feeling and response create each other ceaselessly. When the principle of feeling and response has been developed to the most refined and delicate state, then it can be applied inexhaustibly for practical use. The first step of Pushing Hands practice is to give special emphasis to the training of feeling and sensibility. When one's feeling and sensibility are ingenious and alert, the changes (i.e., one's changing responses to situations) will be fine, delicate, and inexhaustible.

Dialogue

When I question, he answers. One's question and the other's answer produce movement. When there is movement, the substantial and insubstantial will be clearly differentiated. When practicing Pushing Hands, I detect with my mind and question with my energy. After he answers, I then "hear" or perceive his substantial and insubstantial aspects. If there is no answer to my inquiry, then I can advance and attack. If he answers, then I must perceive the speed of his movement and the direction of his advance or retreat. At this time I can discriminate his substantial and insubstantial aspects.

Substantial and Insubstantial

When one practices the postures of T'ai Chi, the substantial and insubstantial aspects must be discriminated clearly. For example, when one steps forward with one's left foot, one must first shift one's entire weight to one's right foot, so one's right foot is substantial and one's left, insubstantial—then the movement will be light and nimble. Otherwise the entire body will be clumsy and confused, which is detrimental to health and of no use in self-defense. The Classics say, "The insubstantial and the substantial should be clearly discriminated. Each single part of the body has both a substantial and an insubstantial aspect at any given time, as does the body in its entirety."

When one practices Pushing Hands with a partner, if his body is insubstantial one does not push, otherwise one will fall into his trap. When the opponent's body is substantial one can begin to push, but one must not commit oneself immediately. One must apply the technique called "withdraw and push": withdraw one's hands slightly and then quickly push forward. Only in this way will the push be effective. Otherwise it will be force against force, and the stronger person will win. Hence the Classics say, "If you want to pull something upward, you must first push downward, causing the root to be severed and the object to be immediately toppled." Or, "If your opponent does not move, you do not move. At his slightest stir you have already anticipated it and moved."

"At his slightest stir" means that the opponent's body has become substantial, so before he is able to issue his energy to attack, one takes the opportunity to uproot him while his body is still in a substantial aspect, giving him no chance to counterattack. If his energy has already been issued, one should not counterattack immediately. If one does, it is a collision (again, force against force). Instead, one must adopt either of the two following techniques: 1) Roll Back technique: first yield and neutralize his striking force to the side, and then push forward. The "Song of Pushing Hands" says, "Entice him to advance; when his energy is emptied, adhere to him and issue energy." When beginners practice Pushing Hands, they must learn this well. 2) Receiving energy: When 70 percent of the opponent's entire striking force has been issued, utilize the remaining 30 percent of his force which has not yet been issued to counterattack. If one can apply this technique correctly, one's opponent will be pushed far, far away. One will then have reached a high level of T'ai Chi.

In the T'ai Chi Classics it is said, "The energy when mobilized is like steel refined a hundred times over. There is no stiff [substantial] adversary who cannot be overthrown." The way to discover the insubstantial and substantial aspects of an opponent's body is to practice Pushing Hands with feeling and sensibility, "hearing" the opponent's energy. The insubstantial and substantial aspects are so important to the student that I must repeat my explanations again and again in order to arouse the students' special attention.

Taking the Measure of the Opponent

The *Art of War* says, "If you know yourself and know your opponent, in one hundred battles you will have one hundred victories." Therefore, before marshalling and marching the army, one should first examine his own troops and take the measure of the enemy, estimating the conditions of victory or defeat. How true this is! The origin of victory or defeat lies in knowing or not knowing. Although in comparison with military affairs boxing is a trifling matter, its principles are all the same. To meet the other's excellence with one's own defects is called miscalculation; to meet the other's defects with one's own excellence is called a clever strategem. The way of gaining victory is a matter of clever strategy on the one side and miscalculation on the other. Therefore, taking the measure of the opponent is of the utmost importance.

That which is called the "dialogue" of T'ai Chi is inquiring about the opponent's movement in order to perceive the direction and center of gravity of his energy. This is examining the opponent's condition and is called "taking the measure of the opponent." Before either side has advanced to attack, I should meet action with tranquility and meet his strenuous exertion with a leisurely attitude, and without the slightest preconception. "If the opponent does not move, I do not move; at his slightest stir, I have already anticipated it and moved beforehand." The really important point is that during the one movement of contact between both sides, I immediately know his substantial and insubstantial aspects and how to deal with them. All of this comes from feeling and sensibility, "hearing" energy, substantial and insubstantial, dialogue, and taking the measure of the opponent. The student should pay careful attention and devote all his energy to acquiring this art.

Note—Those readers interested in pursuing the principles in the above paragraph more deeply are referred to the most profound and famous of Chinese treatises on military strategy, Sun Tze's *Art of War.—Ed.*

To Know Before the Action

"Before the action" means that Yin and Yang have not yet separated. It is utterly infinitesimal, almost nonexistent. To perceive this moment is called foreseeing. It has no sound, no smell, is formless and bodiless. When one puts (this technique) to functional use, one must apply it during the time when no movement or definite posture has yet occurred (i.e., the opponent is just about to move, but has not yet moved). Thus, he has no opportunity to use his techniques. All those whose art has reached the highest level can predict the action. If one knows before the action, he can make a superior position of his own. This is called, "From nothingness something is created" and "Seize the opportunity to act." Those whose art is on a low level know nothing about foreseeing the action, and thus cannot obtain a superior position of their own. The way of T'ai Chi can be divided into three levels: that of one who has foresight and vision; one who knows and apprehends only after the event; and one who knows nothing from beginning to end. As soon as fellow disciples of T'ai Chi join hands and begin to practice the Pushing Hands exercise, they can perceive each other's level of mastery. It is not necessary to decide by actual combat. It is like playing chess. When a highly skilled player makes any move, it is meaningful and foresighted and hits the mark. The conditions for victory or defeat have already been determined. The moves of a player of lesser skill are superficial and shortsighted; he has no purposeful idea in mind before moving and so is not able to gain the upper hand. He plays into the hands of his opponent and is unable even to look after himself. It is apparent that he is doomed to defeat. The principle of Pushing Hands is the same. When it is performed by a superior person, his mind is tranquil, his ch'i is sunken, and his postures are elegant and graceful. He can meet an adverse situation by yielding without hitch or hindrance and can apply his technique at will in a natural way. The person of lower skill finds himself in a dilemma—able neither to advance nor retreat. There is no strategy for defense or offense. This is all due to whether or not one can "know before the action."

Double-Weighting

Double-weighting means the absence of substantial and insubstantial . . . The T'ai Chi Classics say, "When the weight is kept sunk on one side, your postures will be compliant and agile; if double-weighted, the postures will be clumsy and stagnant." Again it says, "The reason that even one with several years of practice of this art cannot apply it for practical use and is generally subdued by the opponent is that he has not yet comprehended the defect of double-weighting." The defect of double-weighting is very difficult to apprehend and comprehend. Unless one knows the principle of substantial and insubstantial, he will find this defect unavoidable . . . In Pushing

Hands practice, when the opponent pushes me with all his might, if I resist with force against force, it is a collision and is called stagnation . . . If I do not use force against force, but follow the opponent's incoming force while inducing him to advance, not resisting and not letting go, then his energy will come to naught. This is the result of keeping the weight sunken on one side. The Classics say, "Diligent practice brings the skill of interpreting (hearing) energy."

To Give Up Oneself and Follow the Other

To give up oneself and follow the other means to give up one's initiative motion and follow the movement of one's opponent. In the art of T'ai Chi it is a matter of utmost importance because as soon as two persons join hands ready to engage in combat, with a serious attitude toward winning or losing, and neither wants to yield or forego his rights as he attacks, they will soon discover that that which is called "giving up oneself and following the other" is not merely a literary explanation, but contains very profound significance in the art of T'ai Chi. The student must study diligently to cultivate his Nature. The Classics say, "T'ai Chi is evolved from Wu Chi; it is the origin of motion and tranquility and the mother of Yin and Yang." Motion and tranquility are the Nature; Yin and Yang are the principle. The Nature and the principle are the source of the Way. The student must constantly devote effort to cultivate his mental faculties (i.e., his Nature) and study hard, examining subjects thoroughly, in order to comprehend with the mind and apprehend with the spirit. After a long time, it will suddenly dawn upon him. The Classics say, "Diligent practice brings the skill of interpreting energy; beyond this achievement lies the ultimate goal, complete mastery of an opponent without recourse to detecting his energy." This is the principle of advancing by orderly stages . . . When one's technique becomes so fine and delicate that one can create a superior position of his own and a defect in his opponent without worrying about not being able to get a superior position or create a defective position for the opponent, one will have reached the stage in which one can yield everywhere at the opponent's slightest pressure and adhere to his slightest retreat. Thus, one will hold an advantageous position no matter what one is facing—this is called "giving up oneself and following the other."

Stimulation

Sinking the ch'i, relaxing the waist, emptying the abdomen, holding in the chest, pulling up the back, slumping the shoulders, lowering the elbows, stretching and expanding each joint comfortably, combining all the energies of motion and tranquility, insubstantial and substantial, inhaling and exhaling, opening and closing, yielding and unyielding, leisurely action and rapid action—all these are called "stimulation." When the mind mobilizes the intention, when the intention mobilizes the ch'i, and when the ch'i mobilizes the body (circulates throughout the entire body), then the energy of stimulation, which is latent within, will be created. When the mind and ch'i are joined and linked together with the variations of substantial and insubstantial, the energy becomes so very strong and fast that it is like a howling typhoon and fearful waves, or passing clouds and flowing waters, or a flying hawk and a leaping fish, or a hopping rabbit and a swooping falcon, now sinking, now rising, suddenly appearing and suddenly disappearing. The stimulation of the natural greatness of the ch'i is inscrutable like the winds and clouds.

The technique of Pushing Hands is to utilize the energy of stimulation to shock the opponent, causing him to be like an ocean liner caught in a storm, thrown in and out of the billowing waves. He falls down from dizziness, helpless as a baby. My center of gravity is difficult to detect. This is the function of stimulating the energy.

Foundation

To practice the postures of T'ai Chi is good for health and to practice Pushing Hands, Ta Lu, and the T'ai Chi Dance is good for practical use. When one first practices the postures, laying a proper foundation is of utmost importance. In practicing the postures, one must seek correctness and exactness. Each posture must be central, upright, tranquil, and comfortable. The movements must be slow, light, agile, rounded, and lively. This is the way to enter the gate. The student must follow the proper sequence and make gradual progress so that time and effort will not be spent in vain and he can acquire the art in the shortest way.

Centrality means that the mind and the ch'i are centered and harmonized; the spirit of vitality is clear, and the ch'i sinks deeply to the tan t'ien. The root is in the foot; this is the foothold. The center of gravity is in the waist and spine—this is what the Classics mean by saying, "The source is in the waist." The spirit of vitality is concealed within and not exposed without, then one can have central equilibrium and deep tranquility.

Upright means that the postures must be correct and proper and must avoid leaning or inclining . . . When issuing energy or extending and aiming in a certain direction, you must maintain your center of gravity. For the center of gravity is the axis of the entire body. When the center of gravity has been firmly established, the movements of opening and closing will be alert, active, and at will. If the center of gravity is not well established, then the opening and closing loses its pivot point. It is like an axletree of a cartwheel; if the axletree is not on center and is not adapted to the center of gravity of the cart, then the turning of the cartwheel as it goes forward or backward will lose its usefulness. When the postures are correct, the center of gravity will be secure . . .

Tranquil means peaceful, quiet, and relaxed, avoiding any tension. Obtaining peace and tranquility in a natural way so that the ch'i can circulate throughout the entire body with no impediment comes from the peaceful and secure postures, the even and regulated movement, the deep and slow respiration, and the calm ch'i and spirit of vitality.

Comfortable means stretching out comfortably. Therefore the Classics say, "At first seek open and expanded postures; later seek to make them close and compact." When one first practices the postures, the movements should be open and widely stretched, enabling every section of the joints to be comfortably expanded. One must not intentionally use external muscular force to expand the sinews and bones, but make the movements in a natural, slow, and relaxed way. With gradual practice, the movements will become relaxed, lively, and sunken deeply.

Light means empty and easy, but not floating. When you practice the postures, the movement should be light, nimble, and slow so that you can advance and retreat at will. Gradually a relaxed and lively energy will be developed. Later the energy of attaching and adhering will be created. Therefore, the word "light" is the first step in practicing T'ai Chi and is the way to enter the gate.

Agile (ingenious) means active and intelligent. From lightness come relaxation and firmness. From relaxation and firmness the ability to adhere and attach will be developed. When you can adhere and attach, you will be able to connect and follow. Only when you can connect and follow will your movement be ingenious and active, so that finally you can apprehend the technique of not letting go and not resisting.

Round means rounded out. The movement of every posture should be rounded out without hollows or deficiencies, so that the whole body can act as one unit and the defects of hollows, projections, and severances will be avoided. When the energy is applied in Pushing Hands practice, it cannot be light and nimble if the postures are not rounded out. If the postures can be rounded out, they will be active. If you can attain roundness in every movement of your postures, there will be no position in which you are at a disadvantage.

Lively means active and alert, without clumsiness and stagnation. If you have a thorough understanding of all the above-mentioned principles, you can stretch and contract, open and close, advance and retreat freely and without hindrance. The Classics say, "If one can breathe properly, one's movement will be agile and active."

To Give and To Receive

The natural temperament of each person is different, and it may generally be divided into two types—the yielding and the unyielding. The disposition of an unyielding person is hasty and ardent. The superior person of this type is stubborn and headstrong, while the inferior is cruel and violent. The stubborn and headstrong likes to contend. Therefore he is inclined to the unyielding aspect when he studies the art of T'ai Chi, because he likes to strive for mastery and, unwilling to submit to others, seeks to outdo them. The disposition of the yielding person is peaceful and compliant. The superior person of this type has the mind and ch'i in coordination and is respectful and magnanimous. His disposition is mostly inclined to the yielding aspect of T'ai Chi because he is peaceful and has much patience. The disposition of a violent person is fierce and rude, so when he starts to learn the art of T'ai Chi he is inclined to furious, quick movements without a delicate and fine tendency. The inferior grade of yielding disposition is weak, has no strong will to learn, and lacks the mind to advance. Therefore when he studies, he does not want to go into details. The true martial arts expert gives importance to an unyielding will (in his own training) and a yielding disposition (toward others). When one possesses wisdom, benevolence, and courage, the hard and soft, substantial and insubstantial will all be in coordination and one can give attention to conduct and enter into studies.

The above mentioned are different types of disposition and are related to the natural temperaments of students. One must heed this well. Owing to the different temperament of each person, his achievement will also vary. We have often observed that even disciples who learn from the same teacher vary in their postures and explanations of the principles, and thus leave many doubts and misunderstandings. Therefore the teacher must suit the teaching to the different dispositions of the students, and the slightest divergence will take one far from the path. So I am here to make this clear in order to elucidate doubts as a means of reference.

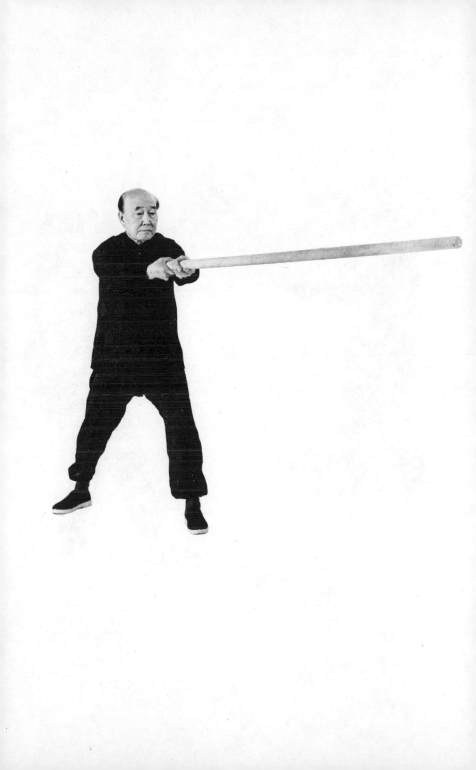

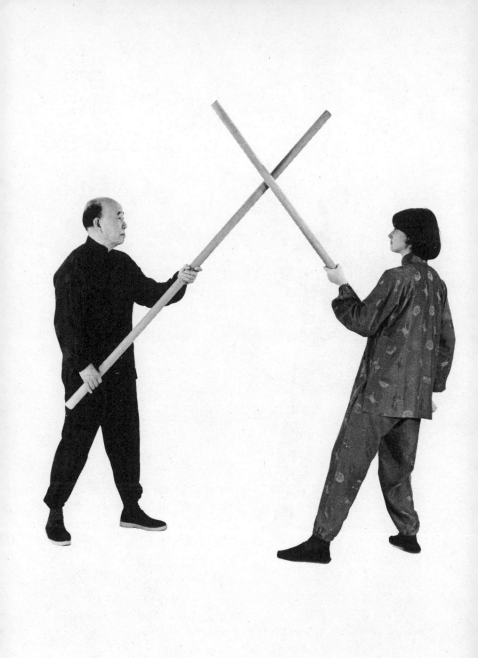

14
Stories of the Masters

● The deflection of a thousand pound momentum
by a trigger force of merely four ounces and an
old man's defeating great numbers of young ones

In the T'ai Chi Classics, it is said: "There are many different
schools of the martial arts. Although their forms and styles
differ, they can never go beyond reliance on the strong taking
advantage of the weak, of the swift conquering the slow.
Hence, they represent purely natural physical attributes, and
are not related to the techniques discussed later. Strength and
quickness cannot explain, and have no part in, the deflection
of a thousand pound momentum by a trigger force of merely
four ounces—or an old man's defeating great numbers of
young ones." When one's skill in T'ai Chi has reached a high
degree, one achieves the invaluable technique of inducing the
opponent to attack and then neutralizing his attacking force in
such a way that he becomes powerless. He cannot use his
energy, even though he may possess a striking force of a thousand pounds.

Formerly, west of Peking, there lived a rich man named

Chang who owned many houses and whose farmstead was as large as a city. He was addicted to military pursuits, and had thirty resident boxing teachers. On learning of the outstanding reputation of a great T'ai Chi master named Yang Lu-chan, of the Kuang Ping Prefecture, he entrusted his friend Wu with the mission of inviting the great master Yang to become his private teacher.

When the great master arrived at his house, Chang observed that he was a short, thin fellow, plainly and simply dressed and of not very attractive appearance. Because of this appearance, Chang slighted him and treated him with small courtesy, and the feast provided for the teacher was less than abundant. The great master, understanding the reasons for this, poured his own wine and drank alone, as there was no one near him. Chang was displeased by this behavior and said: "I've often heard Mr. Wu mention your famous name, but I don't know whether T'ai Chi can be used to strike a man."

The great master Yang replied: "Only three kinds of men may not be struck." Chang then asked: "Who are they?" The great master answered:

"1. Men made of brass.
2. Men made of iron.
3. Men made of wood.
Besides these, there is no difficulty."

Chang said: I have thirty good boxers in my house. Instructor Liu is the best among them, and is capable of lifting a weight of five hundred catties [pounds]—can you do combat with him?

So they stood up and started to spar. Liu's striking postures were as ferocious as a tiger's and his fists were as swift as a whirlwind. When his striking fist got close to the great master, Yang neutralized the striking force by turning his body slightly to the right; the force of the stroke was dissipated and rendered powerless. He then patted Liu lightly with his left hand, and the instructor fell away more than thirty feet.

Chang clapped his hands, laughed, and said: "What an inscrutable art!" Then he gave orders that the food on the table

116

should be removed and a full-course Manchu Chinese banquet brought, for he admired and respected the great master Yang as a teacher.

Although Liu was as strong as a bull, he could not win the bout because he had no techniques. Clearly, the great master won without having a strong physique. Although a man of seventy or eighty is considered old, it is possible for him to defeat numerous men because he knows the techniques of the boxing art. Even though a man is young, it is very hard for him to fight even one or two persons if he has not mastered the art.

When a Chinese general named Hwang Chung, of the Minor Han Dynasty, was not allowed to go to the front because of his old age, he said: "The man is old, but the horse is not old; the horse is old, but the knife is not old." He immediately gave a demonstration of his knife techniques, which were as good as ever. He was then allowed to go to the front and won the war.

When a man practices T'ai Chi, his bones are strong, his blood and ch'i abundant, and his techniques will not diminish even in old age. Although he is old, he is still full of the spirit of vitality; therefore, he can defeat a great number of men.

Master Yang Chien Hou, son of the great master, Yang Lu Chan, once had combat with nine people. They all rushed forward at the same time to encircle and attack him. With several turns of his body, all these people were made to stumble and fall eight to ten feet away from him. Master Yang was nearly eighty years old at the time.

It is not mere foolish talk to say that an old man can defeat a great number of men. Speed or swiftness without technique is mere confusion, not true swiftness, and therefore is of no practical use. Swiftness with technique is true swiftness and can be put to practical use.

● A short biography of the Yang Family

Yang Lu Ch'an was a native of the Yung Nien District, Kuang P'ing Prefecture in Hopei Province. In his youth he traveled to Ch'en Chia Kou in Honan Province to learn the art of T'ai Chi Ch'uan from Ch'en Chang Hsing. Ch'en Chang Hsing stood erect like an ancestral tablet. His bearing, in fact, was so upright that he acquired the nickname "Mr. Ancestral Tablet." At that time all of Ch'en's students belonged to his own clan and no outsiders were permitted instruction. So Yang Lu Ch'an at first was excluded because he was not of the same family, but he was so eager to learn that he stayed on without any rancor or disappointment. Although he lived in the Ch'en village for several years, he received no tutelage. Late one night he was awakened by the sound of training shouts (Japanese *kiai*) coming from an adjoining courtyard. He quickly arose, leapt over the wall, and discovered the building from which the sounds had come. Carefully tearing away a bit of the paper window covering, Yang saw the teacher instructing his students in the techniques of "withdraw and push" and "receiving energy." With great excitement he observed the movements and each night thereafter secretly returned to the spot. Then he would go back to his own room and practice the techniques assiduously. From this time on his art increased greatly.

Some time later Master Ch'en ordered Yang to enter a match against his other students and all of them met defeat at the hands of Yang. Deeply impressed, the old Master considered Yang to be a genius and taught him all his own secret arts. Yang later returned to his native Yung Nien District and began to teach people near his home. Many students came to him to learn. His boxing art became known as "Hua Ch'uan" (neutralization boxing) or "Mien Ch'uan" (flexible boxing) because all of the movements were soft and supple. Subsequently, he went to Pei P'ing (Peking) where he taught members of the royal household and was appointed martial arts instructor to the Manchu Banner Battalion.

Yang's disposition was very forthright and vigorous. He liked to contest with exponents of any other style or school. He would often go about carrying a short spear and a bag, visiting places all over northern China. Whenever he found one whose art was superior to his own, he would ask to test him. Even if the other man would refuse a match, Yang would compel him to contest, but so high was his skill that he would never hurt or injure his opponent. His mastery was such that he was never defeated and he thus acquired the sobriquet "Yang the Unsurpassable."

Old Master Yang was born in the fourth year of Chia Ch'ing of the Ch'ing Dynasty (1799) and died in the eleventh year of T'ung Chih of the same dynasty (1872). He had three sons—the eldest, named Ch'i, died young; the second was named Pan Hou; and the third was named Chien Hou. Each had the ability to hand down his father's art. During the old Master's lifetime many stories about him arose, including the following incidents:

When the Master was in Kuang P'ing he once had a match with a boxer on top of a wall. The man was defeated and was compelled to retreat to the wall's edge. He could no longer stand firmly, his body inclined backward, and he was about to fall down. At this moment of imminent peril Yang suddenly leapt over to the man from thirty feet away and held on to his foot, thus saving him from falling and being killed.

Yang was also very adept at using the shaft of his spear. With a mere flick of his spear shaft he could pick up any light object from the ground. While mounted on horseback, he could shoot arrows without a bow, using only his fingers. Such was his extraordinary skill that he could hit the target every time, missing not even once.

One rainy day old Master Yang was sitting in his hall and saw his daughter ready to enter, holding a brass bowl full of water. When she was just about to step in but had not yet drawn back the screen, her foot slipped on the wet moss near the doorstep and she was on the verge of falling. At this moment the old master flew to the door in one leap, held the bowl with one hand and supported his daughter's arm with the other, saving her from falling. Not even one drop of water was spilled. From this we can see how marvelous was his art.

On another occasion when Yang was fishing on the bank of a river, two famous Shaolin teachers were passing behind him. Ordinarily they feared his famous reputation and did not dare to engage him in combat face to face. Now they perceived an opportunity to push him from behind so that he would fall into the river and drown and his famous name would be sullied. So they secretly agreed to attack the Master simultaneously from left and right. Yang's power of vision was extraordinarily acute and he was aware from the outset that some secret plot was going on behind him. When the powerful striking force of the two men had just about come to his body, he suddenly held in his chest and straightened out his back, using the technique of High Pat on Horse. There was only a slight lowering of his head and rising movement of his back and the two men were propelled together into the river. Then old Master Yang said to them, "Today you are both lucky. If you were on land I would like to use one more technique and then you would not escape so lightly." As soon as the two men heard this they swam speedily away.

One day when old Master Yang had journeyed to Pei P'ing, another famous boxer heard that he was called "The Unsurpassable," became envious, and requested a bout. At first Yang was unwilling, so the other boxer took Yang for a coward and pressed his challenge more vigorously. When it became clear that he could not avoid a bout, Yang agreed. He laughed and said, "Since you are so eager to have a bout, why don't you first punch me three times?" Upon hearing this the other boxer was overjoyed. He raised his fists forthwith and proceeded to strike Yang's belly with all his might. But before Yang's great laugh had quite ended, the other boxer was knocked down and propelled thirty feet away.

Old Master Yang's eldest son, Pan Hou, was born in the seventeenth year of Tao Kuang of the Ch'ing Dynasty (1837). When he was young he began to learn T'ai Chi from his father. Each day he practiced unceasingly, diligently and painstakingly. His father would not allow him to rest even for a short time, and in addition he endured the intolerable pain of being flogged with a whip by his father until he was on the point of running away from home. His temper was irritable and violent; he was very proficient in "free hand" techniques and he enjoyed knocking down his opponents. As soon as he would stretch out his hand, blood would immediately appear from their bodies and some of them would be thrown more than thirty feet away. When Pan Hou was in the prime of young manhood, he once engaged in a match against a famous Shaolin teacher who was very daring and had considerable power. He grasped Pan Hou's wrist and would not let it loose. Pan Hou, using a sudden sharp burst of energy, applied it to the body of the Shaolin teacher. The latter could not stand it and was pushed over. Pan Hou, elated, returned home to give a detailed account to his father. When Lu Ch'an heard the story he laughed and said, "You are happy because you have won. But alas your sleeve has been torn. Can this be called the use of intrinsic energy in T'ai Chi?" Pan Hou looked at his sleeve and saw that it had indeed been torn. He became downcast and withdrew.

He then began to practice T'ai Chi more diligently than ever before and his techniques gradually reached a very high level. It is a pity that he did not wish to transmit his art to many disciples. He was like a singer with a very high vocal range, who could find few to sing in tune with him. So eventually his art became extinct. He died in the sixteenth year of Kuang Hsu (1892).

Old Master Yang's second son, Chien Hou, was born in the twenty-second year of Tao Kuang of the Ch'ing Dynasty (1842). Like his brother, he began learning T'ai Chi from his father at an early age. His father supervised his training with such severity that he was compelled to practice for an entire day without being allowed to rest even a little while. He became so utterly wearied in body and mind that he could hardly stand. Several times he attempted to hang himself, but each time was discovered and rescued. We can see that it was his spirit of enduring hardship at that time that enabled him to make a famous name for himself later on. His disposition was much milder than that of his elder brother Pan Hou, so he had many students. In all he taught three different kinds of postures—higher, middle, and lower. His soft and hard energies in perfect coordination, he achieved the great consummation and his art reached a very high level. When he engaged in combat with experts from other schools who were proficient in using knife or sword, he used only a wooden feather duster to defeat them. As soon as he raised his hand, the opponent's hand would invariably be held fast so that he was put into a disadvantageous position, unable to approach. He could also make good use of the spear shaft. He could issue any kind of energy from the tip of the shaft so that whenever it was touched by the staff of another person the other staff and its wielder would be thrown far away. He could knock a person out with any part of his body and could release all his energy in the moment of a laugh or shout. He was also an expert in shooting "bullets" (spherical iron pellets), and never missed his target. With three or four bullets in his hand, he would often shoot down three or four flying birds. Even more mysterious was his ability to hold a sparrow in his palm without letting it fly away. A bird about to take off must first press downwards with its claws and find a firm foothold upon which to exert energy and raise its body aloft. But Chien Hou could interpret the sinking energy of the bird's two claws. As the bird pushed downward, he would relax and neutralize so the sparrow, unable to avail itself of a foothold, could not fly away. From this we can see that his clever, subtle, and ingenious use of interpreting and neutralizing energy was such that no one else could approach his level. When he was advanced in years, he often practiced to develop his intrinsic energy lying in bed fully clothed. His servants often heard a strange shaking sound at night emanating from the room where he was sleeping.

He died in the sixth year of the Republic of China (1917), a peaceful death without sickness or calamity. A few hours before he died, he received a premonition of his impending death in a dream. He summoned all of his family members and disciples to assemble before him and gave his final instructions to them one by one. After bathing and changing his clothing, he died with a smiling face. He had three sons—the first was named Shao Hou; the second son, Chao Hou, died young; and the third son was named Ch'eng Fu.

Yang Chien Hou's eldest son Shao Hou was born in the first year of T'ung Chi of the Ch'ing Dynasty (1862). He studied T'ai Chi Ch'uan from the age of seven. His disposition was stubborn and unyielding. He enjoyed knocking down his opponents and made good use of free hand techniques, very much like his uncle whose characteristics he inherited. His postures were low and brisk, his movements swift and powerful. In every move he sought compactness. When he taught others he adopted the same style—as soon as he stretched out his hand he would attack. The students for the most part could not stand it, so few remained to learn from him. He had profound skill in "borrowing energy," "sudden energy," "intercepting energy," and "hurling-aloft energy." It is to be regretted that he did not wish to transmit his art to many students, so those who know it are now very scarce. He died in the eighteenth year of the Republic of China (1930). He had one son named Chen Sheng.

Yang Chien Hou's third son, Ch'eng Fu, was born in the ninth year of Kuang Hsu of the Ch'ing Dynasty (1883). His disposition was mild. As a child he showed no great inclination to study T'ai Chi, but at the age of twenty began studying with his father. During his father's lifetime he did not pursue his studies with diligence and his comprehension of the principles remained incomplete and imperfect. After his father's death he suddenly awakened to his responsibility and began to practice assiduously night and day. Eventually he gained a far-reaching reputation. He acquired all of the arts of T'ai Chi, mostly from study on his own. Indeed, he was a marvelously gifted genius. Had he been able to apply his entire mind to study while his father was alive, his achievement would not have fallen short of his grandfather's. His body was stalwart and his stature gigantic; he appeared as soft as cotton externally but internally was as strong as iron. His "withdraw-attack energy" and "receiving energy" were both superb. In contrast to his elder brother he taught most of his students the higher postures so their movements would be wide open and stretched. Because of his mild disposition many students came to him to learn. His reputation spread north and south throughout the country. He died in the twenty-fourth year of the Republic of China (1936). He had four sons—the eldest was named Chen Ming; the second Chen Chi; the third Chen Tou; and the fourth Chen Kuo.

When we speak of T'ai Chi at the present time, we all hold Yang's T'ai Chi in the highest esteem. Fortunately Yang's descendents were all able to acquire the arts handed down by their ancestors and were able to follow in the steps of their forefathers, urging themselves on to efforts so that the fame of Yang's family would be maintained forever.

● The secret bitterness of Yang Family T'ai Chi

How Yang Lu Ch'an compelled his sons to practice T'ai Chi and nearly caused a calamity:

It is well known that Yang Family (i.e., Yang Style) T'ai Chi was developed toward the end of the Ch'ing Dynasty by the great master Yang Lu Ch'an. But the growth and eventual prevalence of Yang's T'ai Chi also contains a secret of extraordinary bitterness and grief.

Toward the end of the Ch'ing Dynasty, after Yang Lu Ch'an had successively defeated eighteen masters of the martial arts in their training halls, he acquired the honorific title, "Yang the Unsurpassable." He then wanted with all his heart to hand down the extraordinary skill which he had spent a lifetime in learning to his two sons Yang Pan Hou and Yang Chien Hou so that Yang Family T'ai Chi could be developed gloriously and brilliantly under his own descendents. With this in mind, Yang Lu Ch'an adopted a training program of unprecedented severity in supervising his two sons' practice of this art. Frequently he knocked his sons down, causing their heads to bleed and their mouths to be split open. Under this severe training, the two sons met with unspeakable suffering. One must realize that, although a martial arts man may say that all depends upon painstaking and hard practice, natural talent is also an indispensable ingredient. Pan Hou and Chien Hou, under their father's strict supervision, met with unbearable bitterness in their training. What the two sons found most difficult to bear was their father's insistence that they practice according to the maxim, "For ten years one sits near the window (studying), not allowing eyes to stray even once to the garden." Lu Ch'an did not allow his sons to take even one step out of the family courtyard; they were to remain at home training day and night. One might well ask, how long could two youths in their prime endure such treatment? The result was that Yang Pan Hou once scaled the wall and escaped, but was intercepted and brought back. Yang Chien Hou tried to hang himself, but was rescued. Only after these two calamities did Yang Lu Ch'an come to realize the (correct) way of practicing martial art—each one has his own natural talent, and progress cannot be forced. So he could do nothing but become a bit more lenient in his supervision.

But Yang Lu Ch'an had also admitted several "outsiders" as his personal disciples. Of these, the senior named Chen Hsiu Feng had attained the highest standard in the art. Just because of this, several incredible and unexpected events took place.

Chen Hsiu Feng, Standing in Front of Yang's Tomb, Usurps the Title of Head Disciple:

In 1872 Yang Lu Ch'an became ill and died and was brought to his native place for burial. His two sons and disciples carried his coffin to the hillside cemetery. When the coffin of the great Master of his generation had been lowered into the ground, the senior disciple Chen Hsiu Feng suddenly stood up before the tomb of his deceased teacher and before the earth had even dried he declared, "Yang's T'ai Chi is no longer in the hands of his descendents!" As soon as the words were out, everyone was startled. Chen Hsiu Feng, without politeness, went on to point out that while the Master was alive his two sons had never practiced his art well. Therefore Yang's secret and miraculous techniques had not fallen into the hands of the two brothers; but only Chen Hsiu Feng himself had acquired the Yang family's genuine teachings. Thereupon, Chen Hsiu Feng patted his chest and declared, "I am the only head disciple of the second generation of Yang family T'ai Chi. If there is anyone who is not convinced, please come up and try conclusions with me." Yang Pan Hou and Yang Chien Hou never anticipated that this elder student would snatch away the title of Head Disciple even before the earth on their father's tomb had dried. They were furious and wanted to challenge the elder disciple, but upon considering the matter they remembered that even in daily practice sessions they were no match for Chen. As soon as they practiced with him, they were either knocked out or thrown over. If they were to contest the issue at this time, there would be no advantage whatever. The common saying has it . . . "When the gentleman takes revenge even ten years is not too late." So Yang Pan Hou and Yang Chien Hou endured their shame and anger without saying a word. They merely shot fierce glances at Chen Hsiu Feng, and silently descended the hill.

Hard Practice To Become the Best and Recover Family Fame:

To take up the tale again, when Yang Pan Hou and Yang Chien Hou returned home, they suffered from their inexpressible anger. They also regretted that they had not trained seriously during their father's lifetime because they did not wish to endure the hardships involved. But now they were of a mind to study and practice diligently, so they took out their deceased father's secret manuals and practiced the techniques described in them. The proverb says, "There is nothing difficult under heaven; a persevering will can overcome any obstacle." Accordingly, Pan Hou and Chien Hou, after a period of hard practice, improved their skill by leaps and bounds. After three years they were no longer weaklings, so they went together to seek out Chen Hsiu Feng and challenge him in order to recover by force the title "Yang Family Head Disciple."

At that time Chen Hsiu Feng was teaching T'ai Chi in the Yen Ch'eng district of Honan and had accepted pupils there. Yang Pan Hou and Yang Chien Hou sought him out and found him. After a few cold words of greeting, they came to the point, "Elder disciple, did you not say that the genuine teachings of the Yang Family are no longer in the hands of Yang's descendents?" Chen Hsiu Feng averted his eyes and replied, "Ah, I forget . . . How long ago did I say that?" Chien Hou, seeing that he was feigning ignorance, became very angry and flatly pointed out, "Three years ago, when we carried our deceased father's coffin up the hill and had barely finished burying him, you said those words." Chen Hsiu Feng now put on the appearance of understanding completely and said with a hearty laugh, "Yes indeed! Three years ago I really did say that. But at that time I did it only to intimidate you two brothers to advance. Now all is well; you have practiced hard and after three years, the Yang Family title can return to your hands again."

As soon as he had said this, Chen immediately stretched out his right hand and, lifting the large armchair near him with the sticking energy of his palm, moved it and set it down in front of the two brothers saying, "Very good. You two brothers are not unworthy of being named sons of the great master Yang. This chair can be considered the Head Disciple's Chair. Please sit down." When Chen Hsiu Feng showed off this technique, the Yang brothers looked at each other with their mouths hanging wide open in amazement.

How the Technique of Lifting the Armchair with the
"Sticking Palm" Oppressed the Two Brothers:
The sticking energy of T'ai Chi is divided into three levels—highest, middle, and lowest. A persson with the highest form

of T'ai Chi sticking energy can use his flat palm to lift up anything without exerting any strength through his fingers. In terms of Yang Style T'ai Chi, only this can be called genuine sticking energy. The middle level of this energy is described by the saying, "As soon as one touches his clothing, the opponent is immediately thrown over." That is to say, as soon as your palm touches the clothing of the other man, he is already in your trap. No sooner does your palm touch his clothing than he is thrown over. The phrase used in T'ai Chi practice, "Touching the opponent's clothing, he can be pushed down in (any of) eighteen ways" refers to this technique.

As for the lowest level of technique, it requires that one touch the opponent's body with the hand in order to make him fall, that is, one grasps the opponent's body or limbs. There are two methods. One is borrowing his energy to issue your own energy (receive-attack); the other is to entice the opponent to issue energy, then, after neutralizing, to knock him over. This kind of energy is the most elementary T'ai Chi technique.

Chen Hsiu Feng relied only on the sticking energy of his one palm to raise an armchair of several tens of catties and set it down lightly in front of the two brothers. This highest level of sticking energy even Yang Pan Hou and Yang Chien Hou considered beyond their reach. However, Chen Hsiu Feng's courteous yielding up of the title invisibly relieved the unhappy feeling in the hearts of the brothers, and this can be considered the time when they buried the hatchet and all ended happily.

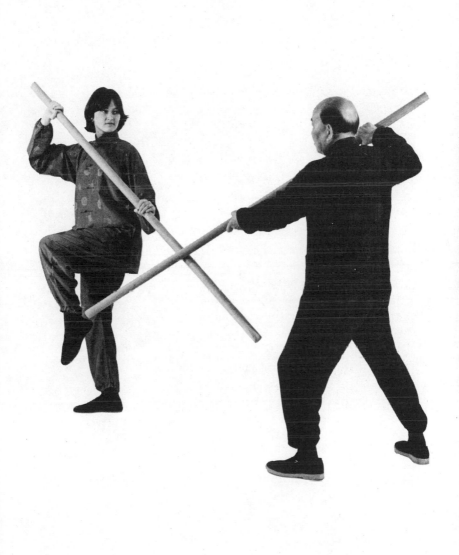

15
Similar Philosophical Points: Lao Tze and T'ai Chi Ch'uan

Lao Tze said: "When the mind rests in the state of nothingness, we can look at the inner enigma; when the mind manifests an inner state of some kind, we can look at the outer aspects."

T'ai Chi: When using the techniques of Adhere, Attach, Connect, and Follow, with no resistence and with no letting go in Pushing Hands practice, we would look at the inner enigma of neutralization; when issuing energy to attack, we look at the outward aspects.

Lao Tze: "Nothingness and something create each other; back and front follow each other . . ."

T'ai Chi: When your opponent brings pressure on your left side, that side should be empty; the same is true for the right side. When he advances, he feels the distance incredibly long; when he retreats, he feels the distance exasperatingly short.

Lao Tze: "The whole universe is like a bellows; it is hollow, yet it is inexhaustible. The more it works, the more comes out of it."

T'ai Chi: The energy appears relaxed, but is not empty. The more pressure you put on me, the more reaction force you will receive (withdraw-attack technique).

Lao Tze: "It is imperceptible and its usefulness is inexhaustible."

T'ai Chi: Outwardly one appears peaceful and quiet, but inwardly one concentrates the spirit of vitality.

Lao Tze: "He chooses to be last and so becomes the first of all. Reckons himself outside and finds himself safe and secure."

T'ai Chi: If your opponent does not move, you do not move; at his slightest stir you have already anticipated it and move beforehand. If you go your own way, your movements will be clumsy; if you give up yourself and follow the other, your movement will be light and alert.

Lao Tze: "When you hold the spirit and the ch'i fast to the body, you can maintain a perfect harmony; when you concentrate your ch'i to the utmost degree of pliancy, it will bring you to the pliability of an infant."

T'ai Chi: From the most pliable and yielding, you will arrive at the most powerful and unyielding. Although the changes are numerous, the principle remains the same.

Lao Tze: "The bent becomes whole; the crooked becomes straight."

T'ai Chi: Seek the straight from the curved; reserve energy before releasing it.

Lao Tze: "When you want to expand, you must first contract; when you want to be strong, you must first be weak; when you want to take, you must first give. This is called the subtle wisdom of life."

T'ai Chi: In practicing Pushing Hands, use the techniques of Adhere, Attach, Connect, and Follow, with no letting go and with no resistance. If he expands, I contract; if he becomes strong, I weaken; when he takes, I give—then I expand, become strong, and take at will.

Lao Tze: "Tao is an endless circle, ever returning."

T'ai Chi: When attacking above, you must not forget below; when striking to the left, you must pay attention to the right; when advancing, you must have regard for retreating —this is T'ai Chi.

Lao Tze: "The softest thing in the world can override the hardest. Such a thing seems to issue forth from nowhere, yet it penetrates everywhere. Again it says, 'Tao does not contend, but it surely wins; it gets responses without calling . . .'"

T'ai Chi: Induce him to advance; neutralize his oncoming force until he becomes powerless, then use four ounces of energy to deflect a momentum of one thousand pounds.

Lao Tze: "The highest form of goodness is like water; in choosing your dwelling, know to keep to the ground. In cultivating your mind, know how to dive into hidden deeps. In making a move, know how to choose the right moment. It is because you do not contend that you will not be at fault."

T'ai Chi: To find out the defects of an opponent and obtain a superior position of your own, conceal your ch'i and spirit of vitality internally and do not expose them externally. The body turns and remains connected (to the opponent), moving neither too soon nor too late. Yield just in time. T'ai Chi is second to none because it does not contend.

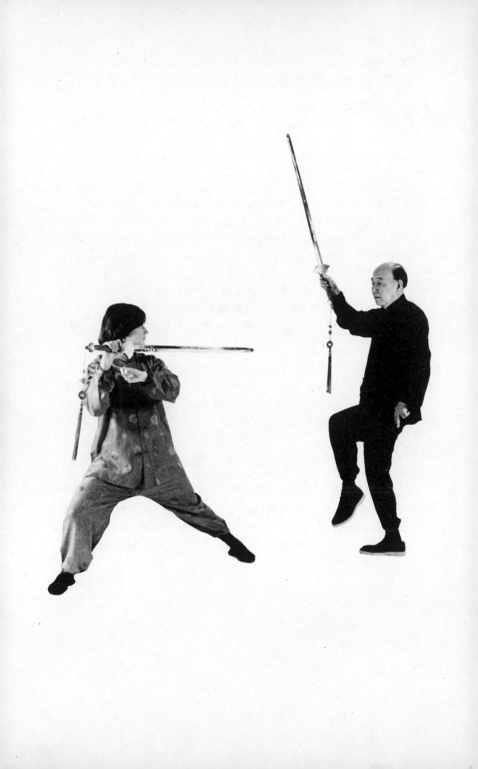

We have so many things worth learning.
But knowledge is unlimited and life is limited.
So even in our whole life we cannot finish our studies.
Life begins at seventy! Everything is beautiful!
Health is a matter of the utmost importance
And all the rest is secondary
Now we must find out how to enjoy excellent health
*   in our whole life . . .*

—T. T. Liang

About the Author

In addition to T'ai Chi, Master T. T. LIANG has studied Shaolin, Ch'in-na, Praying Mantis, and various sword, broadsword, and staff arts. Although his primary interest is in T'ai Chi as a way to achieve health and peace of mind, Master Liang also stresses the importance of knowing the "practical use" of T'ai Chi to attain one's full development in the art. Master Liang taught in the United States for some twelve years, in New York, New Hampshire, and Boston, and he is at present living in Massachusetts.

About the Editor

PAUL GALLAGHER has studied T'ai Chi since 1967 and has been a student of Master Liang's since 1971. He learned Chinese in order to read the original treatises on T'ai Chi and related arts, and has done extensive research on natural healing, diet, and herbs.

VINTAGE ASIAN STUDIES

V-696   **de BARY, WILLIAM THEODORE** / The Buddhist Tradition in India, China and Japan

V-841   **BYNNER, WITTER AND KIANG KANG-HU** / The Jade Mountain: A Chinese Anthology

V-555   **CHOMSKY, NOAM** / American Power and The New Mandarins

V-173   **CONFUCIUS (trans. Arthur Waley)** / Analects

V-843   **DAUBIER, JEAN** / A History of the Chinese Cultural Revolution

V-702   **EMBREE, AINSLIE T. (ed.)** / The Hindu Tradition

V-990   **ENGLISH, JANE (trans.) AND GIA-FU FENG** / Chuang Tsu/Inner Chapters

V-833   **ENGLISH, JANE (trans.) AND GIA-FU FENG** / Tao Te Ching

V-405   **ESHERICK, JOSEPH W. (ed.) and JOHN S. SERVICE** / Lost Chance in China: The World War II Despatches of John S. Service

V-990   **FENG, GIA-FU AND JANE ENGLISH** / Chuang Tsu/Inner Chapters

V-833   **FENG, GIA-FU AND JANE ENGLISH** / Tao Te Ching

V-225   **FISCHER, LOUIS (ed.)** / The Essential Gandhi

V-927   **FITZGERALD, FRANCES** / Fire in the Lake: The Vietnamese & The Americans in Vietnam

V-968   **FRANCK, FREDERICK** / The Zen of Seeing: Seeing/Drawing As Meditation

V-663   **HERRIGEL, EUGEN** / Zen in the Art of Archery

V-244·   **HERRIGEL, EUGEN** / Method of Zen

V-465   **HINTON, WILLIAM** / Fanshen

V-328   **HINTON, WILLIAM** / Iron Oxen

V-610   **HSU, KAI-YU** / The Chinese Literary Scene: A Writer's Visit to the People's Republic

V-841   **KANG-HU, KIANG AND WITTER BYNNER** / The Jade Mountain: A Chinese Anthology

V-708   **KESSLE, GUN AND JAN MYRDAL** / China: The Revolution Continued

V-479   **MALRAUX, ANDRE** / Man's Fate

V-727   **MANN, FELIX** / Acupuncture (rev.)

V-971   **MILTON, DAVID & NANCY AND FRANZ SCHURMANN (eds.)** / China Reader IV: People's China

V-883   **MISHIMA, YUKIO** / Five Modern Nō Plays

V-730   **MYRDAL, GUNNAR** / Asian Drama: An Inquiry into the Poverty of Nations

V-708   **MYRDAL, JAN AND GUN KESSLE** / China: The Revolution Continued

V-793   **MYRDAL, JAN** / Report from a Chinese Village

V-301   **ROSS, NANCY WILSON (ed.)** / The World of Zen

V-303   **SANSOM, GEORGE B.** / The Western World and Japan

V-375   **SCHURMANN, FRANZ AND ORVILLE SCHELL** / China Reader I: Imperial China

V-376   **SCHURMANN, FRANZ AND ORVILLE SCHELL** / China Reader II: Republican China

V-377   **SCHURMANN, FRANZ AND ORVILLE SCHELL** / China Reader III: Communist China

V-971   **SCHURMANN, FRANZ AND DAVID & NANCY MILTON** / China Reader IV: People's China

V-405   **SERVICE, JOHN S. AND JOSEPH W. ESHERICK (ed.)** / Lost Chance in China: The World War II Despatches of John S. Service

V-847   **SNOW, EDGAR** / Journey to the Beginning

V-930   **SNOW, EDGAR** / The Long Revolution

V-681   **SNOW, EDGAR** / Red China Today: The Outer Side of the River

V-945   **SNOW, LOIS WHEELER** / China On Stage

V-411   **SPENCE, JONATHAN** / Emperor of China: Self-Portrait of K'ang-hsi

V-166   **SZE, MAI-MAI** / The Way of Chinese Painting

V-925   **THONG, HUYNH SANH (trans.)** / The Tale of Kieu by Nguyen Du

V-298   **WATTS, ALAN** / The Way of Zen

V-893   **ZAEHNER, R. C.** / Zen, Drugs and Mysticism

VINTAGE WORKS OF SCIENCE AND PSYCHOLOGY

V-286 **ARIES, PHILIPPE** / Centuries of Childhood
V-292 **BATES, MARSTON** / The Forest and The Sea
V-267 **BATES, MARSTON** / Gluttons and Libertines
V-994 **BERGER, PETER & BRIGITTE AND HANSFRIED KELLNER** / The Homeless Mind: Modernization & Consciousness
V-129 **BEVERIDGE, W. I. B.** / The Art of Scientific Investigation
V-837 **BIELER, HENRY G., M. D.** / Food Is Your Best Medicine
V-414 **BOTTOMORE, T. B.** / Classes in Modern Society
V-742 **BOTTOMORE, T. B.** / Sociology: A Guide to Problems & Literature
V-168 **BRONOWSKI, J.** / The Common Sense of Science
V-419 **BROWN, NORMAN O.** / Love's Body
V-877 **COHEN, DOROTHY** / The Learning Child: Guideline for Parents and Teachers
V-972 **COHEN, STANLEY AND LAURIE TAYLOR** / Psychological Survival: The Experience of Long-Term Imprisonment
V-233 **COOPER, DAVID** / The Death of the Family
V-43   **COOPER, D. G. AND R. D. LAING** / Reason and Violence
V-918 **DAUM, SUSAN M. AND JEANNE M. STELLMAN** / Work is Dangerous to Your Health: A Handbook of Health Hazards in the Workplace & What You Can Do About Them
V-638 **DENNISON, GEORGE** / The Lives of Children
V-671 **DOMHOFF, G. WILLIAM** / The Higher Circles
V-942 **DOUGLAS, MARY** / Natural Symbols
V-157 **EISELEY, LOREN** / The Immense Journey
V-874 **ELLUL, JACQUES** / Propaganda: The Formation of Men's Attitudes
V-390 **ELLUL, JACQUES** / The Technological Society
V-802 **FALK, RICHARD A.** / This Endangered Planet: Prospects & Proposals for Human Survival
V-906 **FARAGO, PETER AND JOHN LAGNADO** / Life in Action: Biochemistry Explained
V-97   **FOUCAULT, MICHEL** / Birth of the Clinic: An Archaeology of Medical Perception
V-914 **FOUCAULT, MICHEL** / Madness & Civilization: A History of Insanity in the Age of Reason
V-935 **FOUCAULT, MICHEL** / The Order of Things: An Archaeology of the Human Sciences
V-821 **FRANK, ARTHUR, & STUART** / The People's Handbook of Medical Care
V-866 **FRANKL, VIKTOR D.** / The Doctor & The Soul: From Psychotherapy to Logotherapy
V-132 **FREUD, SIGMUND** / Leonardo da Vinci: A Study in Psychosexuality
V-14   **FREUD, SIGMUND** / Moses and Monotheism
V-124 **FREUD, SIGMUND** / Totem and Taboo
V-491 **GANS, HERBERT J.** / The Levittowners
V-938 **GARDNER, HOWARD** / The Quest for Mind: Piaget, Levi-Strauss, & The Structuralist Movement
V-152 **GRAHAM, LOREN R.** / Science & Philosophy in the Soviet Union
V-221 **GRIBBIN, JOHN AND STEPHEN PLAGEMANN** / The Jupiter Effect: The Planets as Triggers of Devastating Earthquakes (Revised)
V-602 **HARKINS, ARTHUR AND MAGORAH MARUYAMA (eds.)** / Cultures Beyond The Earth
V-372 **HARRIS, MARVIN** / Cows, Pigs, Wars, and Witches: The Riddles of Culture
V-453 **HEALTH POLICY ADVISORY COMMITTEE** / The American Health Empire
V-283 **HENRY, JULES** / Culture Against Man
V-73   **HENRY, JULES & ZUNIA** / Doll Play of the Pilaga Indian Children
V-970 **HENRY, JULES** / On Sham, Vulnerability & Other Forms of Self-Destruction
V-882 **HENRY, JULES** / Pathways to Madness
V-663 **HERRIGEL, EUGEN** / Zen in the Art of Archery
V-879 **HERSKOVITS, MELVILLE J.** / Cultural Relativism

V-566 **HURLEY, RODGER** / Poverty and Mental Retardation: A Causal Relationship

V-953 **HYMES, DELL (ed.)** / Reinventing Anthropology

V-2017 **JUDSON, HORACE FREEDLAND** / Heroin Addiction: What Americans Can Learn from the English Experience

V-268 **JUNG, C. G.** / Memories, Dreams, Reflections

V-994 **KELLNER, HANSFRIED AND PETER & BRIGITTE BERGER** / The Homeless Mind: Modernization & Consciousness

V-210 **KENYATTA, JOMO** / Facing Mount Kenya

V-823 **KOESTLER, ARTHUR** / The Case of the Midwife Toad

V-934 **KOESTLER, ARTHUR** / The Roots of Coincidence

V-361 **KOMAROVSKY, MIRRA** / Blue-Collar Marriage

V-144 **KRUEGER, STARRY** / The Whole Works: The Autobiography of a Young American Couple

V-906 **LAGNADO, JOHN AND PETER FARAGO** / Life in Action: Biochemistry Explained

V-776 **LAING, R. D.** / Knots

V-809 **LAING, R. D.** / The Politics of the Family & Other Essays

V-43 **LAING, R. D. AND D. G. COOPER** / Reason and Violence

V-280 **LEWIS, OSCAR** / The Children of Sánchez

V-634 **LEWIS, OSCAR** / A Death in the Sánchez Family

V-421 **LEWIS, OSCAR** / La Vida: A Puerto Rican Family in the Culture of Poverty —San Juan and New York

V-370 **LEWIS, OSCAR** / Pedro Martinez

V-727 **MANN, FELIX, M. D.** / Acupuncture (rev.)

V-602 **MARUYAMA, MAGORAH AND ARTHUR HARKINS (eds.)** / Cultures Beyond the Earth

V-816 **MEDVEDEV, ZHORES & ROY** / A Question of Madness

V-427 **MENDELSON, MARY ADELAIDE** / Tender Loving Greed

V-442 **MITCHELL, JULIET** / Psychoanalysis and Feminism

V-672 **OUSPENSKY, P. D.** / The Fourth Way

V-524 **OUSPENSKY, P. D.** / A New Model of The Universe

V-943 **OUSPENSKY, P. D.** / The Psychology of Man's Possible Evolution

V-639 **OUSPENSKY, P. D.** / Tertium Organum

V-558 **PERLS, F. S.** / Ego, Hunger and Aggression: Beginning of Gestalt Therapy

V-462 **PIAGET, JEAN** / Six Psychological Studies

V-221 **PLAGEMANN, STEPHEN AND JOHN GRIBBIN** / The Jupiter Effect (Revised)

V-6 **POLSTER, ERVING & MIRIAM** / Gestalt Therapy Integrated: Contours of Theory & Practice

V-70 **RANK, OTTO** / The Myth of the Birth of the Hero and Other Essays

V-214 **ROSENFELD, ALBERT** / The Second Genesis: The Coming Control of Life

V-301 **ROSS, NANCY WILSON (ed.)** / The World of Zen

V-441 **RUDHYAR, DANE** / The Astrology of America's Destiny

V-464 **SARTRE, JEAN-PAUL** / Search for a Method

V-806 **SHERFEY, MARY JANE, M. D.** / The Nature & Evolution of Female Sexuality

V-918 **STELLMAN, JEANNE M. AND SUSAN M. DAUM** / Work is Dangerous to Your Health

V-440 **STONER, CAROL HUPPING** / Producing Your Own Power: How to Make Nature's Energy Sources Work for You

V-972 **TAYLOR, LAURIE AND STANLEY COHEN** / Psychological Survival

V-289 **THOMAS, ELIZABETH MARSHALL** / The Harmless People

V-800 **THOMAS, ELIZABETH MARSHALL** / Warrior Herdsmen

V-310 **THORP, EDWARD O.** / Beat the Dealer

V-588 **TIGER, LIONEL** / Men in Groups

V-810 **TITMUSS, RICHARD M.** / The Gift Relationship From Human Blood to Social Policy

V-761 **WATTS, ALAN** / Behold the Spirit

V-923 **WATTS, ALAN** / Beyond Theology: The Art of Godsmanship

V-853   **WATTS, ALAN** / The Book: On the Taboo Against Knowing Who You Are
V-999   **WATTS, ALAN** / Cloud-Hidden, Whereabouts Unknown
V-665   **WATTS, ALAN** / Does It Matter?
V-299   **WATTS, ALAN** / The Joyous Cosmology
V-592   **WATTS, ALAN** / Nature, Man, and Woman
V-609   **WATTS, ALAN** / Psychotherapy East and West
V-835   **WATTS, ALAN** / The Supreme Identity
V-904   **WATTS, ALAN** / This Is It
V-298   **WATTS, ALAN** / The Way of Zen
V-468   **WATTS, ALAN** / The Wisdom of Insecurity
V-813   **WILSON, COLIN** / The Occult
V-313   **WILSON, EDMUND** / Apologies to the Iroquois
V-197   **WILSON, PETER J.** / Oscar: An Inquiry into the Nature of Sanity
V-893   **ZAEHNER, R. C.** / Zen, Drugs & Mysticism